Hex Strat

# Arts Development in Community Health

# Arts Development in Community Health

## A SOCIAL TONIC

**MIKE WHITE**

*Research and Development Fellow in Arts in Health,*
*Centre for Medical Humanities,*
*Durham University*
*and Senior Research Fellow,*
*St Chad's College,*
*Durham*

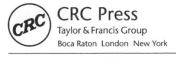

CRC Press
Taylor & Francis Group
Boca Raton  London  New York

CRC Press is an imprint of the
Taylor & Francis Group, an **informa** business

CRC Press
Taylor & Francis Group
6000 Broken Sound Parkway NW, Suite 300
Boca Raton, FL 33487-2742

International Standard Book Number-13: 978-1-84619-140-4 (Paperback)

**Visit the Taylor & Francis Web site at**
**http://www.taylorandfrancis.com**

**and the CRC Press Web site at**
**http://www.crcpress.com**

# Contents

# About the author

**Mike White** is a Research and Development Fellow in Arts in Health at the Centre for Medical Humanities at Durham University and is also a Senior Research Fellow of St Chad's College, Durham. He has over 20 years' experience of managing and researching arts projects addressing community health issues, and he wrote this book with the support of a fellowship award from the National Endowment for Science, Technology and the Arts.

# Acknowledgements

I have benefited from the helping hands and critical eyes of several people. I am grateful to my colleague Jane Macnaughton for spurring me on and to my long-time friends and collaborators Alison Jones and Mary Robson for shared reflection, inspiration and good memory. Mary also did the diagrams for me. François Matarasso mentored me through the draft of the book, and it would have been all the worse, and probably unfinished, without his judicious mix of probing insight and prodding encouragement. Andrew Russell and Phyllida Shaw helped me to think and write better.

In preparing the case examples in the book, I cannot thank the following people enough for their guidance and hospitality: Ann O'Connor in Cork; David Doyle, Lindsay Lovering, Peter Wright and Margret Meagher in Australia; Kate Wells and Peter Stark in South Africa.

I gratefully acknowledge the support and morale boost of a fellowship from the National Endowment for Science, Technology and the Arts, and a visiting international fellowship from Healthway in Western Australia.

My description in Chapter 3 of a music project in an intensive care unit is reprinted with kind permission of Jessica Kingsley Publishers, and parts of Chapter 5 are reprinted with kind permission of DADAA, Fremantle.

First and last, my thanks to Catherine for letting me get on with the research (even during a house move) and to Jonah and Ellie for diverting me from it.

Factors which make for health are concerned with a sense of personal and social identity, human worth, communication, participation in the making of political decisions, celebration and responsibility. The language of science alone is insufficient to describe health; the languages of story, myth and poetry also disclose its truth.

Michael Wilson, *Health Is For People* (1975)

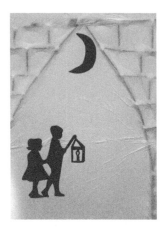

Lantern silhouette. PHOTO: MARY ROBSON

# Introduction

In the last decade health has become a recurrent topic in discussion of the role of the arts in society, fuelled by a growing body of research into connections between culture and well-being. There is now a distinct strand of arts practice that aims to facilitate the experience of well-being among people who are in poor health, or at risk of it, by means of communal involvement in creative activities, and there has been a widespread development of participatory projects addressing health issues.

This pioneering practice of arts in community health, as I shall generically term it, began in the UK in the late 1980s through sporadic pilot projects placing local arts development in health promotion and primary care contexts. It has since grown and expanded to embrace community health on a broad front, hooking up with multi-agency initiatives to address the social determinants of health through partnership working. By 2000, arts in community health had become a recognisable component in the arts infrastructure of the UK, with networks of practice at both regional and national levels.

The rapid growth of this field of work in the UK from the mid-1990s has begun to impact on policy in the arts funding system, on multi-sector partnerships for health service delivery and on local authority cultural strategies. In communities and schools in disadvantaged areas, it has combined creative activities with health education and amassed testimony from participants as to its value. Yet the reasons for the emergence of this field and the nature and diversity of the practice itself have gone largely unaccounted for. So this book considers how and why this field of arts development has come about, the characteristics of its practice and the challenges it poses for evaluation, and it summarises what has been learnt from a number of case studies and other forms of research from the UK and elsewhere.

With support through a fellowship from the UK's National Endowment for Science, Technology and the Arts (NESTA), I have been able to observe the practice of arts in community health and talk with organisers and participants in the UK, Ireland, South Africa, Australia and the United States. It has been possible to undertake at least some preliminary comparison of work in the field across nations with different cultures and healthcare systems in an attempt to locate the well-springs of arts in community health, assess the factors that determine the flow of practice and find some commonality in what those involved in this work are saying about it. I hope to put back what I have taken from these projects by setting out an agenda for meaningful cooperation in research and practice at an international level. I have been further assisted by a visiting international fellowship awarded to me by Healthway in Western Australia to observe practice there in more depth.

There are now many strands of applied social thinking in the UK that have bearing on the development of arts in community health: the 'new public health', the economics of well-being, joined-up government, social value (also termed 'public value'), the active citizenship and social inclusion agenda, epidemiological research on the health effects of self-esteem and status, public/patient involvement in health services, and education initiatives such as the healthy schools standard. These often-interweaving strands suggest to me that arts in community health has not evolved simply as a result of the successful advocacy of an arts sector keen to demonstrate its relevance to health, but rather through the wider recognition of a phenomenological connection between engagement in cultural activity and well-being. It is due to this convergence, and not simply to the debatable effects of the arts acting as a sole instrument to improve health, that some credence can be given to Arts Council England's bold assertion that the arts 'can have a lasting and transforming effect on many aspects of people's lives.'[1]

I refer to the work examined in this book as 'arts in health' simply because that is the term I am most accustomed to using; I recognise that behind phrases such as 'arts for health', 'arts and health', 'arts into health', 'healing arts' and 'arts in health' there can lie different approaches and differing assumptions about the roots of ill health and the ways arts can improve it. The field may, however, be broadly defined as *'creative activities that aim to improve individual/community health and healthcare delivery using arts based approaches, and that seek to enhance the healthcare environment through provision of artworks or performances'.*[2]

Arts in health has become a field of practice encompassing work in hospital acute services, primary care, respite care and rehabilitation, community health and public health, social services and the institutions and contexts where arts therapies are practised, as well as extending across a whole gamut of social policy. The field is now so diverse that we are starting to see some emerging specialities in differing approaches. Some projects may focus on the therapeutic benefits of the arts, some on environmental improvements to support health staff in delivering their care services and some on producing more creative kinds of health information. The capacity-building focus of arts in health work with communities may also be informed by a belief that 'unity is health'. These are arts projects that start from the point of using creativity to enhance social relationships, reflecting growing evidence that good relationships are a major determinant of health. The importance of nurturing and sustaining meaningful human relations in the prevention of ill health has tended to be overlooked in an information society where knowledge may be power but not always be equated with wisdom.

An awareness of the need to mobilise public participation in preventative health strategies that are socialising goes back to the very foundation of Britain's National Health Service (NHS). On the launch of the NHS in 1948, its political architect, Aneurin Bevan, observed:

> The maintenance of public health requires a collective commitment. Preventative medicine, which is merely another way of saying collective action, builds up a system of social habits that constitute an essential part of what we mean by civilisation.[3]

Bevan acknowledged that there is a cultural base to the health service and that we need to make this visible in order for the public to fully engage with it and help shape it. It has taken half a century to realise that participatory arts could have a role in bringing this to light. A commitment to addressing the social determinants of health requires a process of engagement that goes beyond the health services themselves and builds alliances for social change.

Arts in community health is a distinct area of activity operating mainly outside of acute healthcare settings, and it is characterised by the use of partici-patory arts to promote health. The definition of community health I use in this book is a web-based definition found through Google:

> A perspective on public health that assumes community to be an essential determinant of health and the indispensable ingredient for effective public health practice. It takes into account the tangible and intangible characteristics of the community – its formal and informal networks and support systems, its norms and cultural nuances, and its institutions, politics, and belief systems.'[4]

This connects with thinking on 'social capital', which sociologist Robert Putnam has defined as 'social networks and the norms of reciprocity and trustworthiness that arise from them'.[5] The impact of social capital on population health can be significant, as Putnam concludes: '*Positive* contributions to health made by social integration and social support rival in strength the *detrimental* contributions of well-established biomedical risk factors.'[6] Putnam distinguishes between 'bonding' forms of social capital that focus on building cohesion and identity within a closed group and 'bridging' forms that connect different groups together. It has been suggested that participatory arts activity is more successful in building the former type of social capital than the latter.[7] If this is true of arts in community health, it may be due more to circumstance than intent, because the work is small-scale, very localised, targeted to specific communities (often by the requirements of funders) and has only recently begun to achieve the sustainability that can connect projects into demographic or issue-based networks. Social capital theory is problematic in spite of its currency, as I shall explain later, but it helps establish here an important distinction that arts in community health is working in a social model of health rather than a medical one, and its natural allies may be found in the public health arena.

When Richard Smith's editorial in a December 2002 issue of the *British Medical Journal* called for one half of one per cent of the health budget to be diverted to the arts, because 'if health is about adaptation, understanding and acceptance, then the arts may be more potent than anything medicine has to offer',[8] this seemed for arts in health practitioners to be the stuff of dreams. And in dreams it remains. If the shift in funding that Smith looked for had magically occurred, it would have increased Arts Council England's budget by 70%. It would have radically changed our view of the role of art in society, putting arts in health at the forefront of developments in art form practice, their delivery and their engagement with audiences. It is the rationale made for this shift in funding that is most interesting. Smith's use of the word 'adaptation' derives from evolution theory, but more precisely it also looks back to Ivan Illich's affirmation in a *Lancet* article in 1974 that:

> Health designates a process of adaptation. It designates the ability to adapt to changing environments, to growing up and ageing, to healing when damaged. Health embraces the future as well and therefore includes anguish and the inner resources to deal with it.[9]

The consolation of art has often been its ability to support this kind of adaptation at the very edge of human experience. Art can be a potent medium for expressing health – and indeed ill health and distress – and an emphasis on creative messaging is often found at the core of arts in community health, as I believe will be demonstrated in the case examples presented later in this book. Through sustained programmes of participatory arts, shared creativity can make committed expressions of public health, simultaneously identifying and addressing the local and specific health needs in a community. This is what distinguishes arts in health work from art therapies and connects it into social inclusion work. Importantly, this collective action still proceeds from the personal, facilitating engagement by individuals with their own health needs. Arts activity enables a search for meaning and value by and for the whole person and not just for the sick or dysfunctional part. The sharing of health awareness can be both a fact and a metaphor of community arts experience. It is important to not just look at the arts activity in isolation as delivering the benefit; in many instances the benefit can also lie in the quality of relationships forged between arts, health services and other partners such as education, local government regeneration schemes and the voluntary sector.

There is presently a window of opportunity for arts development to help realise a social model of health. The move to multi-agency working is still new to the health services, and the arts can have both an integral and a catalytic role in this. What used to be understood as the preventative approach to healthcare is increasingly about building capacity for change, internally through improved training and holistic approaches and externally in developing social capital. In the light of those observations by Bevan, Putnam and Smith, perhaps it is time to stop arguing for the role of the arts as a useful adjunct to health services and declare that the arts sector, by the very nature of what it does, is in the business of health.

Within the NHS, the operational scale and complexity in delivering the 'business of health' can be daunting for those attempting meaningful engagement with it through the arts. In trying to make sense of local health service structures, a colleague of mine once asked a senior health executive if a map existed of his district showing the boundaries of the various health trusts and the key facilities they governed or influenced. She was told that health trusts and their boundaries had been revised and changed so often in the previous decade that no map was now available, and the information existed, at best, in the heads of those staff who knew the local geography well enough. It seems restructuring is always underway in the health sector, and this anecdote may be indicative of where we are: no longer able to step back and see what we are looking at. So practitioners in arts in community health have had to devise their own 'guide maps' that are both geographically illustrative in building connections between like-minded local projects and temporal in that the continuum of creative health promotion goes from the nursery to the rest home, embraces whole communities and is disseminated as much through celebrations as through health education pamphlets. With a growing intuitive sense of mission, this work has managed to make fair weather through a difficult funding climate.

I will be giving a lot of consideration to the processes of the work, informed by different perspectives and approaches, partly because this is important in understanding how it may be researched and partly because no book has been written on the subject in the UK, so some description of practice is required. The only publications I am aware of internationally on this subject originate from practice in Australia. In particular, I have found parallel threads of thinking to my own in research produced by VicHealth and the Globalism Institute at RMIT University, Melbourne, largely because the practice under review shares many similar characteristics with work in the UK. On the other hand, a book on practice in Australia titled *Promoting Health Through Creativity*[10] is written mainly from the viewpoint of art therapists in institutional healthcare settings, and some of its conceptions of arts in community health seem in my view to be misplaced. It makes the mistake of asserting that well-being is a consequence of creativity. (If it were a consequence, why have so many artists led dysfunctional lives?) What that book does affirm, however, and it is a mutual starting point for my own thinking, is that making art is a biological necessity. At this level there is a fundamental connection to be explored between creativity and health as a pathologically optimistic expression of survival.

Anthropology can provide an interesting lens for examining the effects of arts activities on health promotion and population health. In *Homo Aestheticus*,[11] the US art critic Ellen Dissanayake argues that species-centred art is a behaviour, a biological necessity, which is disciplined by the need to do what feels good in art-making. She considers ritual and art to be socially reinforcing, and that ceremony evolved as a survival mechanism that binds people together. A distinctive quality of art that she terms 'making special' is thus a form of social persuasion, turning what is obligatory for survival into the desirable and addressing substantive communal concerns through evoking deep feelings. These ideas are highly relevant to the practice of arts in community health, though I suspect some palaeontologists and anthropologists might question whether there is the evolutionary evidence to support all her assertions. She refers to 'liminal' transitional experiences producing 'communitas' (the feeling of community). This state of being also relates to Csíkszentmihályi's theory of 'flow', when action and awareness fuse and ego is replaced by a collective sense of 'rightness' that can channel and relieve anxiety or distress.[12] By having control of the process, Dissanayake argues, it becomes possible for participants to speculate and to see the relation of the present ceremony to past and future, a form of scenario building. Dissanayake concludes, 'The reason art is "therapeutic" has at least as much to do with the fact that, unlike ordinary life, it allows us to order, shape and control at least a piece of the world as to do with the usually offered reason that it allows sublimation and self-expression',[13] and she refers to Coleridge in *Biographia Literaria* (1817) on 'the calming power that all distinct images exert on the human soul'. This therapeutic effect motivates participants to repeat the events, creating traditions. They alert us to 'selectively valuable behaviours', so that choice and community go together. Can there then, I wonder, be an alignment between the social determinants of health and the biological determinants of making art? In exploring that question, I intend to make the processes that Dissanayake describes evident in the case examples that are the life blood of this book and to consider what effect they have in generating health awareness and actual well-being within communities.

In the first chapter I will trace the course of the development of arts in community health through the channel of my personal experience in organising projects and discovering the breadth of the field. I look at what has inspired, advanced or sometimes impeded this development and at the challenges it poses for research.

In Chapter 2 I consider how the new public health's goal of addressing the wider social determinants of health has evolved and how this sets a context for arts in community health to help achieve effective communication and engagement with the public. I look at a growing concern in the health sector for meaningful community engagement and consider how creative approaches can be developed to achieve this. I explore whether there is now an underlying philosophy in public health that is of direct relevance to participatory arts activity and whether it offers an effective framework for joint practice. I then look at the current vogue for considering social value and an economics of wellbeing as influences on the delivery of health promotion through techniques of social marketing. Evidence-based theories of the impact of health inequalities, societal status and health, and social capital are posited as important drivers of arts in community health and as the basis of a policy arena in which the arts can simultaneously deliver creative health messaging and build social cohesion. I examine what is being done practically to advance the preventative health strategy that is a cornerstone of the government's aim to achieve a 'fully engaged' scenario of public participation in health, as set out in the 2001 Treasury report *Securing Our Future Health*,[14] but recognise the lack of opportunity so far for the arts to engage significantly with this agenda. Finally in Chapter 2 I review the 2007 national arts debate run by Arts Council England to consider whether this helps or hinders the achievement of more mainstream support for arts in community health. This chapter in effect flicks an art pebble across the millpond of joined-up thinking on social policy and examines the extent of the ripple.

Chapter 3 turns attention to the generic qualities and difficulties that delineate the scope of arts in community health and determine its place within the wider arts in health field. I argue that a cross-sector, relationship-based approach to the planning of work and research can unify a diverse range of art interventions in both institutional and community healthcare settings. I consider what is required strategically to address the needs of practitioners in the field, and highlight some shortcomings that impede the delivery and impact of the work. I set out some essential principles that underpin the work and give it a unique identity and vision.

Chapters 4 to 7 present a number of case examples drawn respectively from projects in Ireland, Western Australia, South Africa and northern England. These examples aim to illustrate the points raised in previous chapters. I will look particularly at how these projects reconcile an entrepreneurial approach to the sustainability of their operations with a guiding ethos of community participation and a commitment to mutual care and positive regard. The case examples collectively describe the diversity of practice in urban and rural locations, both building-based and outreach, and a range of target groups and health issues are addressed. These constitute a wide spectrum of possible interventions. This core section of the book attempts to delineate common characteristics of practice, to critically examine what works or does not work and why and to assess how far the arts practice has grounded its thinking in a health agenda – i.e. is it really arts in community health?

Having case examples from overseas allows me to examine how arts in health is applied to community work in other cultural contexts and healthcare systems. How differently is arts in health developed and interpreted, and in what ways is it a globally shared experience, particularly in relation to public health? The common ground in this work will be identified, with consideration of whether an international research agenda can be articulated and shared. I decided not to pursue case examples in the United States, as arts in health there currently seems very much dominated by arts in hospitals and care institutions, although there are isolated instances of community-based projects. Through social networking, the US produces large collaborative artworks addressing health issues, such as the awe-inspiring AIDS quilts, but I could not see these as being 'community-based' as defined in this book.

Chapter 8 deals with the burden of proof. It examines the problems and obstacles for effective evaluation and producing persuasive evidence of impact. It considers how and why social projects are problematic for evaluation in public health and the additional difficulties the arts bring to collecting viable data and testimony for qualitative evaluation that is more than just anecdotal evidence. A key consideration is how quality in the arts activity itself and in the experience of participants can indicate therapeutic or social benefits. I will assess some frameworks and models for evaluation of community-based arts in health, partly based on the trial-and-error experience of projects to date. This chapter will pose some fundamental research questions for practice and how they may be best addressed.

The final chapter is a casting of bread upon the waters. It considers how cross-disciplinary practice and research could be strengthened through the field of medical humanities and speculates on what it is that sustains arts in community health even when it lacks a favourable policy environment. It takes views from professionals and academics in a range of disciplines that connect with public health and community development. Interview excerpts gather opinion on what the aims, process and outcomes of arts in community health should be.

I have chosen to subtitle this book *a social tonic* for two reasons. Firstly, I consider how participatory arts can be an enlivening social manifestation of health in communities. Secondly, within a musical metaphor, I am looking at how a multi-sector engagement with communities through the arts can establish a tonal centre that entrains a range of interventions to 'sing from the same sheet' as regards community health development.

I have made several journeys in the course of writing this book, through memory, literature and landscape. I put myself into the book as a traveller rather than as an expert, and hope that what I have observed, learned and discussed in the field can adequately set out for practitioners of arts in community health the authenticity of their work and its challenges and achievements and offer a route map for future connections.

## REFERENCES

1 Arts Council England. *Ambitions for the Arts.* London: Arts Council England; 2003.
2 CAHHM. *Determined to Dialogue: a survey of arts in health in the Northern and Yorkshire regions.* Durham: University of Durham; 2002.
3 Bevan A. Quoted in *The Report of the Chief Medical Officer's Project to Strengthen the Public Health Function.* London: Department of Health; 2000. p. 4.
4 Portland State University. *Research Guide for Community Health.* Available at: www. lib.pdx.edu/guides/resources.php?category=15 (accessed 29 July 2008).
5 Putnam R. *Bowling Alone: the collapse and revival of American community.* New York: Simon and Schuster; 2000. p. 19.
6 Ibid. pp. 326–7.
7 Cave B, Coutts A. *Health Evidence Base for Mayor's Cultural Strategy.* London: East London and City Health Action Zone; 2002.
8 Smith R. Spend (slightly) less on health and more on the arts. *BMJ.* 2002; **325**: 1432–3.
9 Illich I. Medical nemesis. *J Epidemiol Community Health.* 2003; **57**: 919–22.
10 Schmid T, editor. *Promoting Health Through Creativity.* London: WHURR Publishers; 2005.
11 Dissanayake E. *Homo Aestheticus: where art comes from and why.* Seattle: University of Washington Press; 1992.
12 Csíkszentmihályi M. *Creativity: flow and the psychology of discovery and invention.* New York: Harper Perennial; 1996.
13 Dissanayake, op. cit. p. 83.
14 UK Treasury. *Securing Our Future Health: taking a long-term view* [the Wanless Report]. London: HM Treasury; 2001.

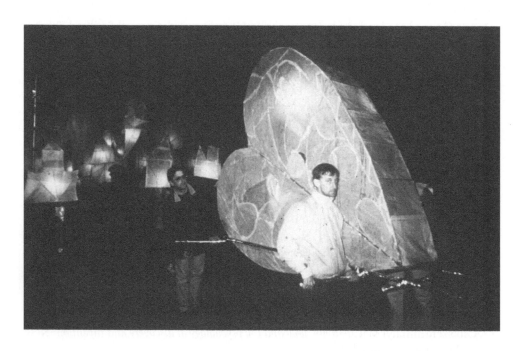

Gateshead *Happy Hearts* lanterns. PHOTO: SHARON BAILEY

# CHAPTER 1

# A story so far

## OUT OF AFRICA

To get to the Siyazama doll-makers' village in Msinga, you take the urban highway north out of Durban to Pietermaritzburg and then travel an ascending road through sugar cane fields to Graytown. From there you enter an arid high valley of baked red soil peppered with thorn bush and aloes.

This journey (in August 2006) is punctuated with reminders of the HIV/AIDS epidemic in KwaZulu-Natal, where one in five people is infected, perhaps amounting to as much as one in three of the sexually active population. Along the way, the car passes a number of white stone circles where Shembe abstinence ceremonies are performed, and the road's verges are interspersed with provincial government billboards exhorting 'Condomise!'

This is my second visit to South Africa in a year to learn about the Siyazama rural crafts project, which aims to promote HIV/AIDS awareness. The project's manager, and also my host, is Kate Wells of the Design Department at Durban University of Technology. Siyazama means 'we are trying' in Zulu. Back in Durban I saw the banners for the project's exhibition at the University of Michigan; the exhibition had an accompanying strapline to its name that translates as 'together we can make a positive difference'. At Msinga I am to see at point of origin how a traditional tribal craft is being reworked and revitalised to express health messages and also provide the education and economic opportunities of a genuine cottage industry.

Despite Lobolile Ximba's 'live' directions over a cell phone, Kate is unsure where exactly to turn off the road (though she has been here many times before). Just as she is about to u-turn, she spies Lobolile by the side of the road waiting for us in her best clothes. Warm greetings are exchanged. She gets into the car and we head off down a long rugged gully. Eventually crossing a dried-up riverbed, we can see beyond the opposite bank the huts of Lobolile's village rising through the dusty heat. Lobolile proudly shows us the home she has had built on the proceeds of Siyazama – £600 will buy a lot in Msinga. All around the walls of the adjacent workshop – also newly constructed from sales income – are arranged dolls in various stages of fabrication and in sizes varying from pepperpot to near life-size, some already adorned with the encrypted beadwork that carries the health message.

We have brought cooked chickens and bread for lunch. 'Gogo' (Granny) has walked the 10-mile round trip to the nearest store to bring the best grape juice. We are shown into the communal cooking hut – it is impeccably clean but sparse, and there are tribal talismans hung over the door. A crumpled HIV/AIDS poster is on the rear wall. 'For the children really,' one mother tells me later, 'as we adults are mostly unable to read or write.' Some of the women have put on traditional Zulu dress for our visit, their red circular headdresses making them appear strangely madonna-like in the interior half-light. A visibly sick mother and child shuffle past us as we enter but return later redressed for the social occasion that I had not anticipated our visit would be.

After lunch, down by the kraal I interview Lobolile and two other women via the student interpreters who have come up with us from Durban. The doll-makers have lived with the daily debilitation of HIV/AIDS infection in their community. Their village is at the epicentre of an epidemic, and the sickness is as pervasive as the red dust that blows around their homes. There are not many men around in Msinga; most are migrant workers in the city. On their infrequent visits home to their wives, they are reluctant to 'condomise', as it would appear a breach of trust by either party in the relationship. There is a deep custom-made gulf between health awareness and behaviour change.

The memory of coming out to chat with participants in arts in health work over a village fence in Africa is where I thought I should begin my book. What the women said to me is considered later in the case examples that are at the core of this book. The conversations I had with them against the wide horizon of a nation in health crisis led me to feel I had journeyed to the interior of arts in health practice – because although this is a place of sickness and poverty, there is also hope in the evident signs of a revitalised cultural tradition linked to health awareness and the self-esteem that comes from gainful occupation. The Siyazama craftswomen are indeed trying to break down the cultural stereotypes that make them vulnerable to HIV infection, and their dolls are silent provocations for the need for change in relationships and sexual behaviour.

Neighbourliness is at the core of all this. As Gogo said to me, 'When you look at your neighbour a metre away and you're doing the same thing and you talk about AIDS, if you say something and one person doesn't understand it, you explain it to each other and you can then explain what you feel about it.' Siyazama is not an atypical example of how creativity can be applied to community health development. While the health issues and cultures may differ, there is in the approach much similarity with projects in the UK and elsewhere. Community-based arts in health is becoming a small-scale global phenomenon. What has resonated for me from this observational visit in South Africa is that there is a fundamental social connectivity in the application of participatory arts to the promotion of community health. To explain this, I need first to consider the origins of community art in Britain and to retrace my own experience of its development in a community health context.

## A NEW ALLIANCE FOR COMMUNITY ARTS

How and where did an alliance between the arts, public health, and education sectors begin in the UK? I believe it can trace its roots back to the community arts movement that emerged in the late 1960s in terms of both the techniques and approaches that have been developed. Adrian Henri's *Total Art*[1] tracks the development of performance art from the 1920s onwards and shows how, despite its esotericism, this connected with the emergence of community arts in the 1960s. Henri says of this kind of art intervention in public space that 'it is not meant as information but as experience', and he observes, 'If England has made a contribution to this genre, it is in the area of social involvement.'[2] These art-oriented social projects originated in provincial rather than London contexts, and they came from an urge to use environmental forms to bypass the modern tradition of the isolated artist.

Though there may have been a distinctly English provincialism in the emergence of socially engaged community art, it nevertheless drew on international currents of radical thinking that challenged the role of art in society and the educationally aloof realm of commodified high art. As long ago as 1934, the US educationalist John Dewey had declared in *Art as Experience* that:

> The values that lead to production and enjoyment of art have to be incorporated into the system of social relationships. The hostility to association of art with normal processes of living is a pathetic, even a tragic, commentary on life as it is ordinarily lived. Only because that life is usually so stunted, aborted, slack or heavy laden is the idea entertained that there is some inherent antagonism between the processes of normal living and creation and enjoyment of works of aesthetic art.[3]

For Dewey, the hegemony of the art market had made the communication of creative impulses esoteric and elitist. He saw this as having both a mental and physical effect on the vitality of the nation. Although the division that Dewey deplored between art and ordinary living appeared most acutely within American capitalism, in Britain it had insinuated itself into the aestheticism of the late Victorian era and also into the self-help tenets of industrialism. Nineteenth-century enlightened capitalism that expounded the educational virtues of the arts for the masses, as exemplified in Mathew Arnold's *Culture and Anarchy* (1869), maintained a hermetic seal on the potential of arts to be socially engaged beyond intellectual improvement and refinement of feeling. A bourgeois belief that art should incite admiration as the proper channel of civilised engagement with creativity still held sway at the foundation of the Arts Council of Great Britain in 1947, despite the influential contemporaneous writings of Sir Herbert Read, who argued that the arts are a biological phenomenon with an important social role in human betterment.[4] A state-sanctioned focus on education through art mitigated the kind of raw division that Dewey observed in the US, but it contributed to a post-war public perception of the separation of the arts and sciences, as analysed by CP Snow in *The Two Cultures*.[5] This ideological cultural antagonism has possibly inhibited connections being made sooner between arts practice and a social rather than medical model of health.

Theories of informal education developed by the Brazilian Paolo Freire in the 1960s also exerted influence on the participation process of community arts,[6] particularly through the work of another Brazilian, theatre director Augusto Boal, whose 'Theatre of the Oppressed' introduced techniques of interactive forum theatre to explore social and political issues from the standpoint of those affected by them.[7] However, the community arts movement's drive to achieve cultural democracy, with its emphasis on the personal as political, did not at first overtly include health in its vision of the social role of art. The political constructs it placed itself within attempted to define relations of power in art-making but not the relations of health arising from the effects of participatory arts on both individual and communal well-being. From the 1970s, some community artists who were disillusioned with this moved into the field of art therapies in order to professionalise their interest in the psychological impact of arts practice. Potential early pioneers were thus lost to another discipline, and community arts may consequently have missed an early opportunity to engage with an emerging question in health thinking as to who and what should define health.

Owen Kelly's seminal work *Community, Art and the State*[8] traced the original impulse of community art in Britain to a desire for cultural activism that could liberate people to gain control over some aspects of their lives, but he also identified dilemmas of practice that are still largely unresolved – tensions that have dogged the development of arts in community health over the question of whether it is an agent of social transformation or a mere instrumental tool. Kelly held it to be the first duty of community arts practice to resist state control, as its destiny lies in the transformation of society, opening up 'a process of co-authorship, of collectivity, underlying all creative activities . . . we have created means where people may combine the roles of producers and consumers, enact these roles socially and collectively, and move as a group towards competence and community.'[9] It is a pity that Kelly's Marxist polemic does not pause to unpack his language. It is tantalising to think that an aspect of 'competence' might relate to health, though Kelly does not say so explicitly.

The rough-and-ready iconoclasm that came stereotypically to define community arts practice from the mid-1960s tended on the one hand to an enforced populism by practitioners ('let's free the people through art') and on the other to the quality-conscious reserve of the art establishment in accepting community arts as the illegitimate offspring of the fertile performance art movement that Henri describes. A Thirty Years War in the arts world about process versus product begins here.

The resonance of an insurgency of socially engaged arts, particularly in the field of theatre, was eventually recognised by the Arts Council in its 1984 review *The Glory of the Garden*.[10] Although this policy document led to an unwieldy two-tier funding system and was maligned at the time as an exercise in cost-cutting rather than a genuine redistribution of funding, it was nevertheless a wake-up call to the geographic and ethnic diversity of arts development in Britain. It took another 10 years for the physical infrastructure that was lacking for its support to be provided through the National Lottery.

Another driver towards arts in community health was the SHAPE network developed by Gina Levete in the late 1970s and early 1980s, which brought arts access issues into the health and social services arena from the perspective of service users themselves. Although ostensibly a loose federation of arts and disability agencies across the UK, some local SHAPE projects also engaged with mental health services and care homes for the elderly. SHAPE East Midlands, for example, in the late 1980s developed arts projects expressing clients' views on the shift of services for people with mental health problems from institutional support to care in the community. The North East's Artists Agency collaborated with Northern SHAPE in 1988 in setting up the Sunderland Art Studio, modelled on an earlier hospital-based project at Cherry Knowle in County Durham, which provided opportunities for mental health service clients to work alongside professional artists in an open studio environment. Also, the Manchester Hospital Arts Project founded by Peter Senior in 1973 established a satellite organisation called START in 1985 to provide arts in non-institutional settings for mental health patient referrals. This helped to produce a wider pool of artists with experience of working in non-hospital healthcare environments.

The earliest instance of community-based arts in health to the best of my knowledge is in the health promotion events at the 1984 National Garden Festival in Liverpool, instigated by the city's (then) director of public health, John Ashton. At this event, music and poetry figured in the 'spot check' health tests offered to visitors. Reflecting on this some years later at the UK's first international arts in health conference in Manchester in 1999, Ashton observed that through the Garden Festival's regeneration programme:

Connection began to be the order of the day, with the reintegration of the humanities into the practice of technocratic public health. The work began to shape up as a combination of agenda setting, consciousness raising and developing models of good practice. In all of these an eclectic approach and a recognition of the importance of connecting to cultural influences and understanding and implicitly drawing on the arts was already apparent.[11]

Through Liverpool's involvement in the World Health Organization's Healthy Cities initiative launched in 1986, Ashton developed a lifelong association with poet and painter Adrian Henri. For example, in 1997 Henri curated an art exhibition on public health for the 150th anniversary celebrations of the city's public health service; this was part of a wide-ranging arts programme 'to help stimulate a consciousness about what public health actually is.' Ashton's pamphlet *Esmedune 2000*, influenced by William Morris' *News From Nowhere* (1890), set out his dream for public health in Liverpool. In it he says:

> We had learned that the public frequently has a much better instinctive understanding of the real issues underlying health than have many health professionals; that the public is much more ready to recognise that health services are just one part of a canvas dominated by issues of economics and development, culture, knowledge, skills, power and control.[12]

The broad canvas that Ashton sets out, however, belies indications that the effectiveness of community-based arts in health is actually in its ability to be up close and personal. Relationship-building in both individual projects and networks is at the heart of this work, often guided by reflective practice on how we can connect and work together, not just what we do to address local health needs. The personalised approach has been important for two reasons: firstly, because community-based arts in health has always been driven by its local champions; and secondly, because it has evolved through, or even in spite of, the rapid pace of change within health services themselves. Not that the arts sector has been stable either, and its funding system has until recently only tended to regard arts in health as a peripheral if worthwhile activity. So the individual relationships of entrepreneurial enthusiasts from different sectors have had to stand in for a strategic partnership.

## BEGINNINGS OF A JOURNEY

As so much of this book is written from my firsthand experience of projects, I think I should explain how and why I personally became involved in arts in community health, the key things I have learned from it, and the challenges I see that it poses for research and evaluation.

What initially sparked my interest in this work was a randomly chosen book on community health and a conversation with a maverick GP, both events occurring on the same day in 1987. That year I was living in South Cumbria and working for Welfare State International, the world-travelled celebratory theatre company whose influential work has been widely acclaimed and documented.[13] The company, which was formed at that seminal time in the late 1960s when performance art and community arts converged, devised vernacular ceremonies, civic spectaculars and handcrafted transitional images whose aesthetics aimed to reconnect people to their landscape, history and popular culture, and to each other. In the late 1980s, the company was working on a three-year arts development programme in Barrow-in-Furness at a time when the Trident submarine construction programme there was at its peak. The giant construction sheds made the terraces and tenements of Vickerstown look from a distance like an industrial Lilliput. Becoming increasingly aware of the stresses that the 'nuclear deterrent' industry's dominance placed on the community, I was interested to engage with local health issues but could not make the right connections. I felt I probably needed a sympathetic health professional to help induct me into a new type of work. So I tentatively looked elsewhere. Someone told me about a Dr Malcolm Rigler in Brierley Hill, West Midlands, who was a fan of Welfare State International's work and keen to have artists working within his practice. I rang him and took up his enthusiastic offer to visit him.

Just before catching a train from Barrow station, I thought I should read something about health on the way down to the Midlands. In a nearby charity shop I found a second-hand copy of *Health is for People* (1975) by Michael Wilson, who, it later transpired, had been Malcolm Rigler's mentor at the University of Birmingham Medical School. This book changed my thinking about and orientation to the role of arts in society. It does not say that much about arts, but it says a great deal about the cultural base of health promotion. I have referred back to Wilson's book many times since. A couple of sentences from it have always had for me the ring of a mission statement:

> Factors which make for health are concerned with a sense of personal and social identity, human worth, communication, participation in the making of political decisions, celebration and responsibility. The language of science alone is insufficient to describe health; the languages of story, myth and poetry also disclose its truth.[14]

Wilson made his life's work an attempt to connect theology and health education, though by the end of his life he had come to feel that 'health education' was a paternalistic and inappropriate term. He preferred to describe it as regeneration work: regeneration not just of social infrastructure but also of individual persons. It was a kind of secular evangelism, which could hold the inherent danger of becoming another form of paternalism, except that Wilson gave primary importance to identifying the 'culture carriers' in a community, who should be at the forefront of a multi-sector approach to addressing the social determinants of health.

When I first visited Malcolm Rigler's Withymoor surgery, I was immediately struck by how small the waiting room was, but it was environmentally welcoming, informative and efficiently organised. His consultancy room looked lived-in and cared for – with books, health pamphlets, plants, toys, snapshots etc. He had even built a makeshift conservatory onto the tarmac car park at the rear. The surgery entrance displayed a prominent and slightly kitsch poster of seagulls with the caption 'Hold on to dreams, for if dreams die life is a broken-winged bird that cannot fly'. He said the words chimed with the feelings of many of his young women patients who were adjusting with difficulty to family life on a large new housing estate where the only point of social contact was the supermarket checkout. The area badly needed a community focus, and he felt the surgery could offer an 'archway' through to a social life on the estate and to discovering the needs and aspirations of its fledgling community.

Malcolm Rigler could see that patients were presenting at the surgery with a great many conditions that were psychosocial in origin. These included depression, stress and broken relationships, which in their turn led to excessive alcohol intake, stomach ulcers, depressed immune systems and added vulnerability to disease. Consequently, obesity, heart disease and unresolved stress were rife. Medical training had not provided him with methods to deal with these problems: 'I was overwhelmed by the great number of conditions I saw for which medical solutions seemed inappropriate. Patients came to me in their droves with problems ranging from divorce to family breakdown to unemployment or post-natal depression, but my medical training had neither prepared nor qualified me for the responsibility of dealing with problems of a personal or a social nature. In its preoccupations with facts and measurements, my medical school had overlooked consideration of an effective communication with patients.'[15]

He saw the solution to this community malaise as requiring the 'prescription of ideas, not medicine'. He embraced the belief of Rev. Dr Michael Wilson that individuals could only achieve true health in a healthy community and that health is not only a private advantage but also a common good. He felt the use of creative arts should figure prominently in his ways of working: 'I always wanted to do all I could to help patients to fully appreciate and understand the fragility and complexity of their own bodies, but I wanted this to go beyond biological facts and simple health education. I believe we could sow the seed of total enchantment with the human, help us all to find a meaning in life and so to value ourselves, our neighbours and the community in which we live.'[16] He had realised that the arts could provide the necessary communication and education with impact, excitement, and insight. We agreed we should find together some small practical means to start achieving this.

I went on to set up with Malcolm Rigler what I believe was the first arts in primary care project in the UK. In January 1988, artists Alison Jones and Art Hewitt spent a week at Withymoor Surgery in a short residency. It was partly research into the potential of arts in primary care and partly a public workshop programme covering activities such as graphics and paper-cuts for waiting room notices, ambient music for the antenatal group and a storytelling evening with the surgery decorated for the occasion. The activities were arranged outside of main surgery times so we would not disrupt the normal working of the practice. Looking back, both the artists and I were nervous, concerned about the appropriateness of our interventions. Nevertheless, there were small, effective outcomes; for example, a workshop making greetings cards to congratulate new mothers was taken up subsequently by practice staff, contributing to an increase in child immunisation from 83% to 98% in a year.

During the residency, Malcolm Rigler arranged for me to visit Michael Wilson at home, now retired, ailing and blind. I vividly remember him sitting by the window against the backdrop of a suburban blizzard, expounding his ideas as the outside world dissolved in a uniform white haze. He spoke of the hierarchical 'war' model of medicine geared to crisis intervention versus the 'peace' model of health in community, and at one point he said, 'I am loath to think of health education work as medicine. It is part of a peace culture, and this development with the arts gives it a new face. Might we call it something new – like regeneration?'

Notwithstanding the 'peace' model, I thought these ideas were explosive, opening a whole new vista for engagement of the arts with community health development. I saw that in the area of health promotion, artists could assist in articulating and making manifest in a caring and concerned way those factors that contribute to the sicknesses of our civilisation – stress, toxins, diet, allergies, drug and alcohol dependency, cancers, heart disorders and AIDS. The arts can develop imaginative educational methods that inform and motivate both the community and individuals to initiate effective self-healthcare programmes. Encouraging lateral interpretation of health themes would give artists a broader social canvas on which to engage directly with the public. It would seem important not just to instil awareness but also to celebrate it.

A key benefit the arts bring is that they may reveal and pronounce our spiritual values and our biological needs and limitations. Unlike clinical medicine, they cannot cure disease, but they can remove unease. Wilson's book showed me that all this was only a step away from the ethos and practice of community arts but gave the field new substance and purpose because 'In community development people are making value choices about what they think makes good community life possible. They share in decisions, they work together to put their plans into effect, and this co-operation in itself is part of what it is to be a healthy community.'[17]

A report on the Withymoor residency was produced for discussion in a seminar hosted at home by the Bishop of Dudley in the spring of 1988.[18] In a belief that this could be a special event articulating a new form of arts practice, Alison Jones spent hours of her own time making hand-sewn invitation cards that would capture the domestic feel of arts in primary care. The seminar brought together local GPs and health service managers, West Midlands Arts officers, the head of the Community College, and another arts organisation with a keen interest in how this project had developed, West Midlands SHAPE.

The seminar paid off, as a few months later Alison Jones was invited to do another short residency at a Midlands surgery in nearby Handsworth, and she then returned to Withymoor to do a longer-term project on the theme of the lungs with the surgery and Thorns Community School. A shed-load of ideas resulted – 3D 'lung boxes', a set of stunning (and punning) posters on all aspects of breathing, a large mobile and a giant banner, all celebrating health in a fun and wildly imaginative way.

The art projects at Withymoor Village Surgery brought people together around non-threatening and enjoyable activities and proved helpful to those who were lonely or suffering from panic attacks or mild to moderate anxiety and depression. The annual lantern procession, started in 1990, was initially conceived as a means of bringing together the socially disenfranchised people of the estate and helping to forge a spirit of community. On its 10th anniversary over a thousand people took part, confirming its success in building community and establishing a tradition.

A list of goals achieved though the use of creative arts with patients at the practice includes: increased access to information, increased understanding of health issues, development of and access to lay referral systems, development of communication skills and confidence, reduction in social isolation, development of a sense of community, increased confidence to tackle causes of ill health, reduced anxiety associated with visiting the surgery, patients' involvement in their own care plans, and improved understanding of patients' own and their community's health needs.[19]

Malcolm Rigler's thinking has particular relevance to current developments in healthcare and health promotion. He has described a blurring of boundaries between what we now think of as physical health, cultural vitality, spiritual balance, quality of life and communal well-being. He argues that we will be seeing a new role for the GP or the pharmacist, who will be less involved with drugs and medicines and will be more of a teacher and stimulator of imaginative solutions. He sees the role of the surgery, in addition to providing personal healthcare, as having a public health function of improving the health of the community:

If we are to improve the nation's health, a key role for a modern general practice team must be to act as an agent for social justice to build opportunities for social engagement through better education and skills training, improved social networks, and meaningful employment opportunities, including voluntary work. My twenty-four years as a family doctor have convinced me that many of the 'medical' complaints reported by patients are in fact the physical manifestations of social, psychological and emotional problems. To create a healthier nation we must start by encouraging inclusive and harmonious relationships in a society where so many find themselves socially excluded. The principal killers are not cancer and heart disease but lack of social support, poor education and stagnant economies.[20]

I can see that Malcolm Rigler has had a profound effect on me and on community artist Alison Jones. Although his idealism could often seem impractical to his peers and even to arts organisations, he was actually quite visionary. He grasped long before I could the potential for arts in health work in new technologies, museum services and public libraries. In speech and manner he had the glazed enthusiasm of a true missionary in a secular world. His commitment to the development of this work ensured that he and practice nurse Lynda Lawley sustained arts projects at Withymoor Surgery until he left there in 1999.

By 1990 Alison had quit Welfare State International to concentrate full-time on this kind of work, and she had formed a partnership with poster designer John Angus working under the name of Celebratory Arts For Primary Healthcare. (Later on, this became Pioneer Projects Ltd, who now run the Looking Well Healthy Living Centre in Bentham – more on that later in the case examples.) And by 1990 I too had left Welfare State International to become arts officer for Gateshead Council on Tyneside. (Sadly, arts in health never took off in Barrow – instead, an arts project developed with a group of local undertakers!) For a while I put on hold my interests in arts in health to concentrate on local arts development and acquiring new skills in managing public art; for example, my work on preparations for Antony Gormley's landmark sculpture *The Angel of the North* (1998), a millennial icon of pathological optimism, began in 1991. As I also became increasingly involved in artwork commissions for local hospitals and primary care facilities, however, arts in health gradually insinuated itself into the core of arts development in a local authority with a poor population health record.

A new opportunity for a community-based arts in health programme presented itself to me in 1992. Gateshead has a higher than average elderly population, and a bid to the King's Fund major grant programme of 1992 on the theme of innovative services for older people resulted in a two-year development grant to set up the Prime Time arts for older people project. The brief was to explore connections between creativity and well-being in later life and address the quality-of-life issue. Prime Time was aimed at active over-60s, but it was run in parallel with an existing council scheme that supported artists' residencies in council care homes. That scheme was managed by Equal Arts, a local arts agency that had emerged out of the SHAPE arts and disability network. It was then possible to have a related arts in health programme extending over the 'third age' and 'fourth age' (age of dependency) and to look at a sample of around 200 Prime Time participants and assess the qualitative benefits that they felt arose from taking part in arts activities. The Carnegie Inquiry into the Third Age, under the chairmanship of former chief medical officer Sir Donald Acheson, published its report[21] in 1993; this report highlighted the connection in older age between positive and engaging leisure time and quality of life, based on research carried out by the Centre for Policy on Ageing.[22]

Prime Time was always focused on project outcomes, represented, for example, by poster poems on Tyneside Metro hoardings, embroidered changing screens for GP consultancy rooms and theatrical tea dance tours. It was a big hit from the start, with all activities fully subscribed. Within a year, a users' forum was coming forward with ambitious project ideas of its own: ideas for animated films including computer animation, woodcarving for public art trails and collaborative projects between art-form groups. The King's Fund's 1992 annual report[23] described Prime Time as a 'delight', and its interim evaluation of the project in that year shored up our confidence that it was developing along the right lines:

> What lessons can be drawn from the experience? That committed, enthusiastic and imaginative leadership creates success. But the paradox is that it is difficult to identify winners like this. It was noticeable during the early stages of the Gateshead project that, notwithstanding the charm of the approach being developed in the project, extreme scepticism was shown about the likely outcomes. Concerns were expressed about keeping the wide-ranging programme under control. Early site visits to the project suggested that the activities were not being carefully appraised. Some of the aspirations of the project (not least, to create the network which is now a major development of the project) appeared to be over-ambitious. These cautions have been overturned one-by-one. The project, very simply, is a story of entrepreneurial success.[24]

In funding terms, Prime Time had an accumulator effect. The King's Fund's programme grant helped unlock business sponsorship and grants from other trusts and from the health authority. By 1993 Prime Time funding exceeded that of the entire arts subsidy we received from the local authority and Arts Council. It became clear that this work could exist outside the arts funding system with a level of public support that made the local councillors feel very comfortable. Validation arguments about the economic importance of the arts became less relevant, because we were seeing the social impact firsthand in the way that scores of older people blossomed. Their TV appearances became matter-of-fact. In 1993 actors from the Royal National Theatre visited Gateshead to read Prime Timers' poems back to them, and in 1994 the group sent its own delegates to speak at a UNESCO conference on ageing in Paris.

The Prime Time musical theatre group toured care homes and day centres on Tyneside. An early production, *It's A Canny Life*, was devised as an interactive soap opera, inviting audience participation in formulating a tale of the effects of alcoholism on three generations of a Geordie family. A key member of the group, a once-housebound lady with a terminal illness, got stuck in the bath one morning. After she was discovered hours later by neighbours, the paramedics were called. Before going to hospital, the lady insisted they take her first to do her afternoon performance in a care home, and would they be so kind as to call back later. This story encapsulates the spirit of enthusiasm and dedication that came to epitomise Prime Time.

Prime Time also opened up opportunities for arts in primary care and health promotion. In 1993 Alison Jones' new company, Celebratory Arts for Primary Health Care, was invited to Gateshead to devise a residency programme leading to finale celebrations for the two-year development period of the King's Fund grant. That summer, an exhibition of the arts in primary care work done in the West Midlands was exhibited in Gateshead Library Gallery, coinciding with a training seminar to launch a new project in Gateshead that would encompass a health centre and nearby schools serving an urban community with high incidence of coronary heart disease. (The public health report for Gateshead in 1992 had noted that the borough had the highest morbidity rate for heart disease in England).[25] The seminar brought together members of Prime Time, local GPs, art workers, teachers and a regional pharmaceuticals representative. The core arts techniques covered included paper-cut decorations and fabric borders for surgery noticeboards and a fruit-sculpture heart, anatomically correct and complete with a pineapple-top 'pacemaker'.

This training session led to a residency at Gateshead Health Centre involving artists Alison Jones and Mary Robson, writer Graham Mort and actor John Flitcroft. They redesigned information display in the practice, and they created large hanging mobiles for the foyer and 3D illuminated heart boxes for waiting areas. Daily displays of fresh-baked sculptural bread provided aromatherapy. Prime Timer Jim Storey, a retired joiner, built a dollhouse terrace of good and bad hearts, displaying in their windows the factors that improve or impair the functioning of the heart. This fascinating and beautiful object was mounted on a surgical trolley and moved around different waiting areas in the practice. Other Prime Timers worked in schools alongside the artists, making 'heart-machines' and 'heart-houses' with local children for exhibition in the clinic. One of these was like a giant Rubik's cube with a different line of poetry on every face;

when manipulated it still produced a logical poem on all sides celebrating the heartbeat (and using a suitable Elizabethan metre!).

By spring of 1994, there were connecting threads of heart imagery running through the entire health centre. Also by this time, pharmaceuticals company Merck Sharp and Dohme (MSD) had commissioned Alison Jones and John Angus to design a series of heart posters with lateral poetic slogans to be printed for national distribution. These posters were devised through feedback conversations with selected Prime Timers who had a history of heart problems. Of the 12 final designs, only one proved contentious with MSD. A Matisse-style dancing figure with the slogan 'Dancing makes the heart grow stronger' was considered 'too soft' by MSD. They insisted on 'Exercise makes the heart grow stronger'. The artists refused. As a compromise, both versions were printed, and a month later MSD agreed that the 'Dancing' version had proved far more popular. This is a classic example of why artists should be trusted to lead the arts in health agenda. Another poster bore the slogan 'Do the rivers run clean in your heart?', connecting individual lifestyle choice to global considerations of ecology and collective responsibility. This image and three others were also printed in large billboard format for the Tyne and Wear Metro, itself a circulatory transport system.

The summation of this project came in the winter of 1994 with Cold Hands, Warm Hearts, a celebratory lantern parade for the Wrekenton and Springwell estates, which are economically deprived areas with a critically high incidence of heart disease. Lantern-making on a happy hearts theme then became an annual event, and from the outset it involved hundreds of local children and their families, voluntary agencies, churches and the area health promotion team. The influence of this project on the development of other health-themed lantern parades in several North of England locations will be explained later in the case examples in Chapter 7. Some of the key principles I learned in the early years of doing arts in community health projects were these:

➤ the role of arts in health in the community is broader than the role of arts in health in hospitals
➤ primary care facilities and the localities they serve should be places where we learn creatively how to be healthy
➤ the arts (and friendly artists) can shape contexts in the community to produce mediating images for health education so that people are 'touched' rather than indoctrinated
➤ the reintegration of art into health checks the dehumanisation of medical science and is essential for both mental and physical health promotion
➤ there is a relationship between creativity and well-being, and to encourage people's latent creativity, community-based arts in health can be domestic, communal, and celebratory.[26]

These seem far less radical statements now than when I first conceived them, but they still affirm for me that this is a new and distinctive area of arts practice, shaping an aesthetic of care from the quality of relationship forged between artist and community. Also, the work grows organically, one project leading on to others as a network is built around the activity. What I became acutely aware of in the early years was that the localised nature of this work was both its strength and weakness, as it was progressing in isolation.

## EMERGING PRACTICE, ADVOCACY AND RESEARCH

By the mid-1990s, I had discovered that there were other beacons out there. There was the ongoing programme of artist residencies at Dr Rigler's practice in Withymoor, and there was Alison Jones' decision to gravitate her work around her home town of Bentham in North Yorkshire, leading to the creation of its Looking Well base. Preston's community arts agency, PRESCAP, had appointed a health and environment worker as early as 1989 to collaborate with the local public health team, particularly on HIV/AIDS awareness. Theatreworks in Sheffield and the Midlands-based THE were developing theatre in health education projects, through touring shows as well as community-based drama residencies. By 1994 Walsall Council's arts team was developing a long-term arts in health programme with local health promotion services and commissioning stand-up comedy shows in workingmen's clubs to promote health issues, accompanied by artist-designed health messages on beer mats. The pioneering holistic approach to community-led regeneration of the Bromley-by-Bow Centre in London's East End had integrated arts into a myriad of services provided to its multi-ethnic constituency. The centre was planning a new health clinic on-site as a prototype healthy living centre. A cluster of arts in primary care projects was developed in Bristol, coordinated by Ruth Hecht. In 1995 Stockport NHS Trust set up the UK's first 'arts on prescription' scheme for GP referrals of people with mild anxiety and depression. Arts Care in west Wales had extended its training work with mentally ill people to address a wide range of socially excluded groups in rural areas whose health is impacted by economic decline. Survivors' Poetry, a self-help group using creative writing, was launched in 1991 by a group of poets who had been through the mental health system, and it eventually grew to a national membership of 2 500. The JABADAO dance company in Leeds had evolved a relationship-based mode of practice in dance and movement work for health with both elderly people in care and under-fives. Characteristic approaches to the work as initiated by these and other organisations will be examined later in Chapter 3 and will be further expounded in the case examples in Chapters 4 to 7.

All of this pioneering work developed more by serendipity than design – projects originated in ad hoc relationships forged with enthusiastic health professionals rather than through cross-sector partnerships, as both health and local authorities were structured at that time literally in divisions.

For most of the 1990s, there was no forum for these fledgling arts in community health initiatives to come together, share their practice and determine the parameters of their work in relation to both arts and health sectors. In 1994 the Calouste Gulbenkian Foundation offered an exploratory seminar for artists working in this new field and also invited public health specialists such as Alex Scott-Samuel from Liverpool to contribute. The following year, the Wellcome Trust convened a wider group of health service managers, researchers, and artists to look at this work as a new field of arts practice. Both seminars were helpful in revealing the impetus to establish community-based arts in health as a distinct current in the arts in health movement – but both foundered on the issue of what would make for useful evidence of the benefit to health services and their users. At that time, projects were individually fuelled by the excitement of breaking new ground in community arts and making what then seemed daring partnerships with health professionals, but there was little sense of there being a collective body of work that could be informed by research. Nor was there an advocacy tool to propagate awareness of the work at national level. An early attempt to provide this was made by the short-lived British Healthcare Arts, a national development agency set up by Carnegie UK Trust, who published a guide to arts in primary care in 1995.[27] This guide viewed the work more as an offshoot of the arts in hospitals field, delivering artworks into other health environments, than as a distinct practice in community health development and health promotion. Yorkshire Arts' 1996 publication *Serious Fun*,[28] however, pointed up a range of arts practice in its region that addressed the social determinants of ill health through what it termed the 'logical link' of arts, primary care and health promotion. Eventually, in 2002, Arts Council England (ACE) would produce a CD-Rom and brochure on the breadth of arts in health practice as an advocacy tool directed to senior management in NHS trusts.[29]

In 1996 the King's Fund gave artist John Angus a grant to produce a research report on community-based arts in health.[30] This is one of the earliest papers to consider this field as an area of research, and interestingly it is written from the viewpoint of an arts in health practitioner. At that time it seemed there was no body of research available that John Angus could refer to, so he undertook to begin an appraisal of the work from his own vantage point as an artist and to examine the appropriateness of a range of evaluation methodologies used in the health sector. It should have been an influential document, but it sold poorly.

At the end of the 1990s, it took the King's Fund to provide the diversifying arts in health field with an umbrella organisation that could give it a collective voice. A consultative report commissioned from Phyllida Shaw[31] identified the need for a representative body for arts in health and motivated the King's Fund's grants director, Susan Elizabeth, to raise the resources for setting up the National Network for the Arts in Health (NNAH). From the outset, the NNAH director, Lara Dose, dealt even-handedly with claims on her attention from arts in hospitals and community-based projects, providing the unifying voice needed for effective political influence. The NNAH achieved membership of around 500 in its first year and set about assembling an archive of information resources to support its advocacy work.

The tipping point, for me personally and I believe for the arts in health field in general, came with the two Windsor conferences held in 1998 and 1999.[32] These were organised by the Nuffield Trust with the (then) chief medical officer for England, Sir Kenneth Calman. They brought arts practitioners from acute hospital and community settings together with the deans of the major medical schools, health researchers and social entrepreneurs. The communiqué that issued from the second Windsor conference on arts and humanities in medicine in 1999 stated that:

> Whilst social and other health scientists have demonstrated various positive correlations in this area, the underlying causal mechanisms remain to be explored. The link between art and health is now recognised to be a social process requiring new and fundamental research.[33]

An outcome of the Windsor seminars was the setting up in 2000 of the Centre for Arts and Humanities in Health and Medicine (CAHHM) at Durham University, where Calman had taken up the post of vice chancellor. This research centre has aimed to meet the groundswell of interest from many areas of social policy and academic disciplines in the importance of the arts as a force for improving the health and well-being of communities and individuals. CAHHM has worked with government departments such as the Department for Culture, Media and Sport, the Department of Health and the Social Exclusion Unit, as well as with the Arts Councils of Scotland and England; and with policy 'think tanks', producing evaluations, briefing documents and literature reviews in the field of arts in health. The centre also builds multi-sector sub-regional networks of arts in health practice, assists research-guided programme development done by clusters of individual projects, mentors individual artists in reflective practice on their work and conducts multidisciplinary evaluations of hospital arts programmes. On the medical humanities front, the centre's director, Dr Jane Macnaughton, runs the personal and professional development strand of Durham's medical school curriculum, and with the professor of humanities and medicine, Martyn Evans, she has provided editorship of the *British Medical Journal*'s publication *Medical Humanities*. This publication's editorial office was based in CAHHM until 2008. In that year, CAHHM became one of two recipients of major development grants for medical humanities from the Wellcome

Trust (the other beneficiary was King's College London) and was able to focus on developing an interdisciplinary model for scholarship in this field under an umbrella theme of 'medicine and human flourishing'. In 2009, it was decided to shorten CAHHM's title to the Centre for Medical Humanities (or CMH), whilst still retaining its strong interest in the practice and research of arts in health.

In its early years, CAHHM worked to establish itself nationally in the following ways: as a resource for policy-makers in the field of community-based arts and health; as leading research and evaluation in arts in health, particularly articulating its impact on socially excluded communities and groups; and as having a lead role in the development of the new discipline of medical humanities, both in research and curriculum development. The centre runs research and project work in four priority areas: arts in health in community settings, architecture and design of health service buildings, medical humanities, and multi-sector learning programmes in arts in health.[34]

The learning programme eventually became a mainstay of CAHHM's work and assisted the setting up of project work as a precursor to evaluation. It was piloted in a programme called Common Knowledge for Tyne and Wear Health Action Zone in 2000–04. CAHHM has gone on to assist the development of this approach in other UK regions, namely East Midlands and Yorkshire, and in work for the Department of Health on the induction of health trainers. The effectiveness of this approach will be assessed later in Chapter 3, which is on the characteristics of practice.

I joined CAHHM in 2000, initially on a secondment, to help establish its arts in health portfolio, but I then decided to stay on. In some respects it offered a natural continuity from my work in Gateshead, but what attracted me was the opportunity to still be connected with on-the-ground practice while at the same time exploring in an academic environment the issues that arts in health poses for effective research and evaluation. Other UK academic institutions have also become engaged in this inquiry. Peter Senior's Arts for Health consultancy moved into Manchester Metropolitan University in the mid-1990s. The Sidney de Haan Research Centre was established in 2002 at Canterbury Christ Church University, developing a speciality in research on singing and health and establishing in 2008 the first international academic journal of arts in health, published by Routledge. Its inaugural issue includes an overview of arts in health in England.[35]

A growing awareness of the complexities involved in finding appropriate means of evaluating the work did not appear to hinder an exponential growth in community arts projects addressing health issues. Anecdotal evidence of successful arts interventions in health attracted the notice of the first term of the Blair government in the *Policy Action Team 10 Report*, which viewed participatory arts (along with sport) as a potential means of tackling social exclusion.[36] The millennium marked a time when significant engagement with the arts by the health sector emerged through several of the health action zones and healthy living centres that had been set up to tackle health inequalities. A statement on healthy living centres issued by the Department of Health in July 1998 recognised that 'mental health is as important as physical health and the imaginative use of the arts can be important.'[37] Although this is sloppily worded – it could imply that the arts assist mental health issues alone – it was still at the time an unprecedented call for a creative partnership. It seemed amazing that arts proposals for major health initiatives were at last being welcomed, and quickly. My own experience of getting arts projects written into the Tyne and Wear Health Action Zone suggested the initiatives were timetable-driven and more about bid culture than a well-considered cultural bid. There was little spare money, however, in the arts components of these development projects to fund the kind of research that would reach the significance required for publication in a high-profile medical journal.

In 2000 the Health Development Agency published the first report by a health organisation into community-based arts in health.[38] The report's researchers identified over 200 community-based arts in health projects going on in the UK in 1998. The questionnaire survey that was the basis of their report produced 90 responses from community-based arts in health organisations, an 'overwhelming' number of which identified improvement in mental health. There was observational evidence of participants achieving stress reduction (53% of projects), therapeutic benefit (57%), improved sociability (59%) and skills development (70%). The survey also highlighted the development of interpersonal skills (72%), opportunities for making new friends (64%) and increased involvement (57%) as being amongst the most important contributions to intermediate indicators of health improvement that an arts project can make. The most common funding sources for the work were local authorities (53%), charitable trusts (50%) and regional arts boards (43%). Only a handful of projects received funding directly from health service budgets, however, indicating the work was far from becoming mainstreamed within the health sector. This may also explain why the researchers were unable to obtain comparative data on health service reductions elsewhere or on quantified savings as a result of arts interventions. Forty-nine per cent of projects revealed they had a budget level under £20000.

The questionnaire returns later formed the core of an online projects database developed by the National Network for Arts in Health. This included financial information on projects, though analysis of that data, to make cost comparison with other kinds of intervention for example, was again not undertaken.

The report noted that around half the projects surveyed were attempting to carry out evaluation formally or informally but that there were 'no established principles and protocols for evaluating outcomes, assessing the processes by which outcomes are achieved, and disseminating recommendations for good practice.' The report, however, identified three emergent approaches to evaluation:

1 *health-based approaches* testing what the arts contribute to self-esteem and their effect on qualitative self-assessments of well-being
2 *socio-cultural approaches* derived from recent assessments of the social impact of the arts
3 *community-based approaches* adapted from social capital theory on health improvement.[39]

In the report, the 'overwhelming' number of projects that identify improvements in mental health suggests that arts interventions in this area could be at the core of research and practice in arts in community health.

The UK government's Social Exclusion Unit produced a *Mental Health and Social Exclusion* review in 2004 that called for a strengthened evidence base to enable the wider roll-out of arts interventions, as they are 'believed to have a therapeutic role as well as helping people reintegrate into wider society by increasing self-esteem, confidence and social networks'.[40] CAHHM was commissioned to do a literature review on arts and adult mental health[41] for the community participation strand of this report. In the report's action plan, the Department of Health and the Department for Culture, Media and Sport proposed jointly to commission research (in a first-time collaboration) to establish the health benefits and social outcomes of participation in arts projects and the characteristics of effective practice. This two-year study was led by Anglia Ruskin University with the University of Central Lancashire, using a common methodology with a sample of projects representative of the scope of practice, and with a range of measures enveloped in 'a theory of change' approach.[42] This was possibly a more qualitative study than the government departments had hoped for, but it facilitated real engagement between researchers and the researched.

## POLITICAL DEVELOPMENTS – AND SETBACKS

By 2003 it seemed that a momentum was picking up for a breakthrough in the mainstreaming of arts in health work. The policy 'think tank' ippr (Institute for Public Policy Research) was asked to arrange a series of Whitehall seminars on the social impact of the arts, leading to the publication *For Art's Sake?*, to which CAHHM contributed.[43] Also in that year, the Smith Institute organised a seminar in Downing Street showcasing work by clients in ACE's social exclusion portfolio – presentations were given on the Creative Partnerships arts in education initiative, on arts and criminal justice work and on CAHHM's involvement in arts in community health. As local authorities began to take the central role in local strategic partnerships to deliver health and care services, the Local Government Association highlighted the importance of arts in health for local cultural strategies[44] and in its long-term vision for mental health services.[45]

In the space of five years there had been three major international conferences on arts in health representing the broad gamut of practice: in Manchester in 1999;[46] at the European arts in health forum in Strasbourg in 2001,[47] where the UK secretary of state for culture, Chris Smith, emphasised the importance of arts in health in developing the cross-cutting agenda for social inclusion at both regional and national level; and in Dublin in 2004.[48] Most of the keynote speeches at these conferences, however, said little about the social context for arts in health in the wider agenda of social capital and community regeneration, and they spoke mostly from the healing experience of arts in healthcare settings rather than the health promotion dimension of arts in health in community contexts.

By contrast, in February 2001 at a health action zones national conference in Newcastle organised by CAHHM, the (then) secretary of state for health, Alan Milburn MP, said, 'I believe the arts can play a very, very important role in ensuring those messages about healthy lifestyle, and about engagement between services and the communities they serve, can be enhanced.'[49] This statement highlighted the government's increasing concern to rebuild trusting relationships between the NHS and the public, recognising that effective communication on health goes far beyond clinical and environmental dimensions. The health action zones opened up a field for arts interventions in health that was wider than had previously been thought possible, and they could move evaluation issues out of the rather narrow and tricky framework of assessing health gain through clinical outcomes to a more holistic assessment of the contribution of community development to fostering human relations and a culture of care in health services.[50]

On the public health front, with the advent of a national consultation in 2004 leading to the strategy publication *Choosing Health*[51] and to a new public health bill, national public health conferences in the UK had arts as an integral strand of their programmes. Also in 2004, ACE announced it was working on a national arts in health strategy. In the following year, the Department of Health announced a review of arts in health, and in inviting responses was deluged with information, including many evaluation reports, from over 300 organisations across the country.

There were helpful indications at this time that key decision-makers were prepared to sidestep the complexities in the evidence issue and look at the broader social benefits for health that arts might bring. This was evident in late 2004 when Liverpool, flushed with its success in acquiring a European Capital of Culture designation, hosted a 'Health and Arts Think Tank'. Here, ACE's chief executive, Peter Hewitt, focused on workforce development issues in both the arts and health sectors and on social-value-oriented research into the emotional and psychological impact of the arts as a precursor to health improvement. The (then) arts minister, Estelle Morris MP, said the arts in health field did not need to produce hard clinical evidence – the case for arts in health made sense – but asked how it could be sold to the public and have its momentum become irreversible as government returned to focusing on human values in healthcare rather than technology and infrastructure. These statements gave rise to some optimism that the validation of arts in health could come in a culture shift and not just a body of evidence from scrutinised projects, and that Liverpool had the opportunity in 2008 to be in the vanguard of this change through its Creative Communities programme.[52]

Then, unexpectedly, things took a downturn in 2006. Health action zones had been wound up, and some of the first wave of healthy living centres faltered into non-sustainability. The senior civil servant who initiated the Department of Health review of arts in health resigned in the face of a troubled financial out-turn for the NHS after several years of unprecedented growth. The ACE strategy and the Department of Health prospectus for arts in health were delayed in publication, largely due to disquiet about possible adverse press reaction. With financial pressures upon it, ACE axed several arts in health clients as casualties of an across-the-board decision to remove 'regularly funded organisation' status from clients receiving less than £20 000 a year. A 'downsizing' of ACE's central office resulted in the removal of its arts in health officer post, and while its newly established Sustainable Communities unit offered some prospect of channelling support for community-based arts in health, it would be likely to do so within a different agenda determined by the Department of Communities and Local Government rather than by the Department of Health.

Worst of all, perhaps, for arts in health practitioners, the national representative body NNAH, having exhausted the charitable trust support that provided a third of its needed income and with cash-flow problems looming, decided to go into dormancy in 2006, suspending its role in providing an independent and unifying voice for the field. This occurred at a crucial time when several regional or issue-based arts in health networks supporting local practice were expressing interest through ACE in coalescing into a national 'network of networks' in tandem with NNAH.

Some momentum appeared to be restored again in early 2007 with the joint publication by the Department of Health and ACE of *A Prospectus for Arts and Health*.[53] This was a far more upbeat, glossy document than had been anticipated, though to a cynical eye it looked like 'feel good' advocacy was replacing any move for a 'cash on table' strategy. The prospectus was launched shortly after the government announced that £675 million of lottery funding would be diverted in order to pay for the 2012 Olympics, and few realised how quickly and painfully the cuts would start to bite. Only days before the prospectus's launch, it had been revealed that ACE's Grants for the Arts scheme, a principal source of funding support for arts in health, would suffer a whopping 35% cut.

This cut meant that during the funding year 2007/08, only £54 million would be awarded, down from £83 million in the previous financial year. Henceforth, arts in health projects would be competing alongside many other calls on this funding from across the arts sector in a much smaller pool.

Despite an untimely launch in a dire funding climate for both the arts and the health service, the prospectus offered some ground for cautious optimism. In particular, the Department of Health's background document to the prospectus, *A Report on the Review of the Arts and Health Working Group*,[54] was robust and positive in its key findings, which are as follows:

> ➤ arts and health are, and should be firmly recognised as being, integral to health, healthcare provision and healthcare environments, including supporting staff
> ➤ arts and health initiatives are delivering real and measurable benefits across a wide range of priority areas for health and can enable the Department and NHS to contribute to key wider government initiatives
> ➤ there is a wealth of good practice and a substantial evidence base
> ➤ the Department of Health has an important leadership role to play in creating an environment in which arts and health can prosper by promoting, developing and supporting arts and health
> ➤ the Department should make a clear statement on the value of arts and health, build partnerships and publish a prospectus for arts in health in collaboration with other key contributors.[55]

The original remit of this review was circumscribed to the role of the arts in healthcare environments, therapies and workforce development. Perhaps due to the wide-ranging submissions and evidence the review received, the final report acknowledges that the arts also successfully support both the department's and the government's objectives in the public health arena. Importantly, this was the first official endorsement of arts in health by the Department of Health, and speeches at the publication's launch made clear it was to be the first step in influencing opinion for cross-departmental support for the work.

Compared with the report and the prospectus, ACE's own publication, *The Arts, Health and Wellbeing*,[56] which was launched at the same time, was weak. What in 2004 was promised to be a national strategy was now termed only a 'framework', providing little more than a rehash of the advocacy publications that ACE had produced back in 2002. It would now be up to ACE's regional offices to produce their own action plans for how they might support this work from reduced resources and local partnerships. The problem here is that there are unequal levels of engagement and financial support across the regional offices and that this fragmentation could hinder the development of nationally coordinated programmes of research-guided practice. Although it was gratifying to learn that the Department of Health's review concluded that there is 'a wealth of good practice and a substantial evidence base', it was disappointing that there was nothing in any of these publications to suggest how this might practically be built upon.

At the same time as the Department of Health's review was taking some of the sting out of the evidence challenge, some cultural analysts were beginning to question the claims of arts in health. In 2006 Policy Exchange published *Culture Vultures – Is UK arts policy damaging the arts?*[57] The witty title of this compendium of essays seems unwittingly self-descriptive as a succession of talon-flexing cultural researchers pick away at policy statements and come to the conclusions that the arts sector makes grandiose statements about its role and achievements in delivering social benefits and that it is rubbish at providing any robust evidence base for these claims. It makes for a damning read and could make one wonder if art has any place in addressing social policy issues.

*Culture Vultures'* editor, Munira Mirza, contributed an essay on arts in health that makes useful recommendations in calling for better definition of arts and health and well-being, and for debate by both arts and health sectors on what makes for quality in this work. The real damage in her essay, however, came from an unsubstantiated concern that a process of manipulative social engineering is going on within arts in community health: 'The model of urban regeneration, health and social inclusion that is being developed is "therapeutic" in which social problems become repackaged as individual, psychological problems that require therapy,' from which she concludes: 'they are not about using the arts to express a greater truth about ourselves, but to manage our emotional lives and even perhaps, to placate us.'[58] But since when were social concern and artistic integrity incompatible, and are artists who work with healthcare services so dumb as not to see that they are being used in this way? If, as she suggested, there is a danger of arts 'medicalising' people, how is it that arts in mental health projects are valued most by vulnerable participants because it is the one intervention they feel does not medicalise them?[59] A study commissioned by the UK's Mental Health Foundation showed that people who experienced moderate to severe mental health problems identified the ability to make their own choices and take control as a major factor in the maintenance of mental health.[60]

As to claims that the arts can promote well-being, Mirza points out: 'we might question whether this is as important as other objective lifestyle choices such as diet, exercise, environment, as well as objective social factors, such as the quality and provision of healthcare in the locality.'[61] This misses the point completely. Arts in health, thank God, is rarely 'happy-clappy', and in community-based approaches its practitioners work alongside health staff and other professions to help improve the conditions for lifestyle choices to be self-determined and to make local health services more interactive with their communities. What is happening in arts in community health is not 'social Elastoplast' but a kind of triage to determine what arts interventions are effective in helping sustain healthier neighbourhoods. Maybe artists in this field should try to articulate their own reflective practice more to the public and not leave it to the policy-makers. Many artists have gone beyond simply transposing community arts skills into healthcare contexts; they are developing specific ideas and techniques that are relevant to local healthcare needs, with the involvement of project partners and participants.

The emergence of arts in community health has been fuelled by an aware-ness of the wider social determinants of health, which requires a more holistic approach to health inequalities – which is longhand for addressing poverty. As Indian Prime Minister Atal Bihari Vajpayee once said, 'Poverty is multidimen-sional. It extends beyond money incomes to education, healthcare, political participation and advancement of one's own culture and social organisation.'[62] Community arts cannot solve these problems any more than medicine can, but it can release visions and voices, and it can tool up some people to break out of the kind of poverty that liberation theology describes as the deprivation of any stimulus to change one's condition.

What is worrying is that, just at a time when arts in health is rising up the cultural and political agenda, there are critical vultures swooping to consign it to dead-end arts posturing and policy failure. Those cultural policy analysts who would defend the right of artists to explore and express their worldview seem curiously parsimonious about allowing the engagement of art with health to do likewise.

On the other hand, there was a cogent argument coming forward from other cultural commentators that the 'art for art's sake argument' would not wash anymore and that the social engagement of the arts is essential for affirming their value and understanding their place in human evolution. John Carey's book *What Good Are The Arts?* concludes that we should:

> switch the aim of research in the arts from what critics think to how art has affected and changed other people's lives . . . It needs to link up with sociology and psychology and public health and create a body of knowledge about what the arts actually do to people. Until that happens, we cannot pretend that we are taking the arts seriously.[63]

He sees this problem as arising at the inception of ACE in 1946, when it focused on high art to educate the masses rather than participatory arts. Carey's observations seem prescient in that throughout 2007, ACE conducted a large-scale public enquiry to explore how people value the arts.

Twenty-five years ago, the cultural critic Raymond Williams, in his book *Towards 2000,*[64] predicted that by the millennium the radical means of cultural production in British society would be forced to the margins, but there they would regroup and become mainstream. This rather cryptic prophecy becomes clearer in the context of social exclusion. The margins are not geographical but social – instances of exclusion can be found in most communities. The sheer size and complexity of the tasks at hand with regard to the contribution of the arts in tackling social exclusion will mean that gaps both in practice and in the evidence base are inevitable. As Watt argued in the *British Medical Journal* in July 2001, social inclusion is much more than simply targeting services to certain groups; rather it is a problem for society as a whole:

> Policies to address the problems of target groups are welcome, if they work, but essentially provide micro solutions for a macro problem. Targeting misses large numbers just above the arbitrary threshold. Sinking the iceberg, rather than attacking its tip, is a better basis for public policy.[65]

I would not underestimate 'micro solutions', however; they can inspire others in similar circumstances, and they may be adaptable. There is a kind of universality within arts in community health that connects with Ellen Dissanayake's evolution theory of art-making as a survival reflex to celebrate surplus and 'make special' as a means of affirming social bonding.[66] It is in this anthropological arena that the social determinants of health and the biological determinants of art-making may find common ground.

There are many arts projects throughout the UK that are attempting to establish a continuum of support for people with health problems in order to improve their well-being and creative skills while providing models for social integration. This may inevitably require some preferential targeting of at-risk groups in order to see the 'macro problem'. If harmful cultural habits are obstacles to health improvement, there is all the more reason for pursuing cultural engagement with those whose health is at risk in order to help identify solutions, and arts in community health can have an influential part to play in this. Much of the practice and learning going on in this field can usefully contribute to wider health promotion strategies and the development of participatory arts with the general public. They need not be seen simply as specialist services for an excluded minority, but rather as core applications of the arts to encourage a healthy culture in a healthier nation.

## REFERENCES

1 Henri A. *Total Art: environments, happenings and performance.* New York: Oxford University Press; 1974.
2 Ibid. p. 128.
3 Dewey J. *Art as Experience.* New York: Perigee Books; 1934. p. 27.
4 Read H. *Education Through Art.* London: Faber; 1943.
5 Snow CP. *The Two Cultures and the Scientific Revolution.* Cambridge University Press; 1960.

6  Freire P. *Pedagogy of the Oppressed.* New York: Continuum Publishing Company; 1970.

7  Boal A. *Theatre of the Oppressed.* UK: Pluto Press; 1979.

8  Kelly O. *Community, Art and the State: storming the citadels.* Stroud: Comedia; 1984. p. 137.

9  Ibid. p. 126.

10  Arts Council of Great Britain. *The Glory of the Garden: the development of the arts in England.* London: Arts Council of Great Britain; 1984.

11  Turner F, Senior P, editors. *A Powerful Force for Good.* Manchester Metropolitan University; 2000. pp. 26–8.

12  Ashton J. *Esmedune 2000: vision or dream? (a healthy Liverpool).* Liverpool: University of Liverpool; 1988. p. 9.

13  Coult T, Kershaw B. *Engineers of the Imagination: the Welfare State handbook.* London: Methuen; 1983.

14  Wilson M. *Health is for People.* London: Darton, Longman and Todd; 1975. pp. 59–60.

15  Rigler M. Unpublished briefing paper for Windsor Conference II. London: Nuffield Trust; 2000.

16  Ibid.

17  Wilson, op. cit. p. 38.

18  White M, Jones A. *Celebratory Arts and Primary Health Care.* Cumbria: Welfare State International; 1988.

19  Tones K, Green J. *A Case Study of Withymoor Village Surgery: a health hive.* Leeds: Leeds Metropolitan University; 1999.

20  Rigler, op. cit.

21  Acheson D. *Report of the Carnegie Inquiry into the Third Age.* Dunfermline: Carnegie UK; 1993.

22  Midwinter E. *Leisure Opportunities in the Third Age: The Carnegie Inquiry into the Third Age research paper number 4.* Dunfermline: Carnegie UK; 1992.

23  The King's Fund. *The King's Fund Annual Report.* London: King's Fund; 1993.

24  Brown S. Unpublished evaluation report on Prime Time. London: King's Fund; 1993.

25  Henley DS. *Report of the Director of Public Health 1992.* South Shields: Gateshead and South Tyneside Health Authority; 1992.

26  White M. Art as Health. In: Bruce N, Springett J, Scott-Samuel A, editors. *Research and Change in Urban Community Health.* Aldershot: Avebury; 1995. pp. 401–6.

27  British Healthcare Arts. *Arts and Primary Care.* Dunfermline: Carnegie UK; 1995.

28  Yorkshire Arts. *Serious Fun.* Dewsbury: Arts Council Yorkshire; 1996.

29  Arts Council England. *Arts in Healthcare.* London: Arts Council England; 2002.

30  Angus J. *An Enquiry Concerning Possible Methods for Evaluating Arts for Health Projects.* Bath: Community Health UK; 1999. Republished University of Durham (CAHHM); 2002.

31  Shaw P. *Proposals for the Development of a National Forum for the Arts in Health.* London: King's Fund; 1999.

32  Philipp R, Baum M, Mawson A, *et al. Humanities in Medicine: beyond the millennium.* London: Nuffield Trust; 1999.

33  Philipp R. *Arts, Health and Well-being.* London: Nuffield Trust; 2002. p. 73.

34 Centre for Arts and Humanities in Medicine. www.dur.ac.uk/cahhm (accessed 29 July 2008).

35 Clift S, Daykin N, Camic P. The state of arts and health in England. *Arts and Health.* 2009; 1 (forthcoming).

36 Department for Culture, Media and Sport. *Policy Action Team 10 Report.* Available at: www.neighbourhood.gov.uk/displaypagedoc.asp?id=321 (accessed 29 July 2008).

37 Department of Health. *Healthy Living Centres.* London: Department of Health; July 1998.

38 Health Development Agency. *Art for Health: a review of practice in arts-based projects that impact on health and well-being.* London: Health Development Agency; 2000.

39 Ibid. p. 11.

40 Social Exclusion Unit. *Mental Health and Social Exclusion.* London: Office of the Deputy Prime Minister; 2004. p. 83.

41 Angus J, White M. *Arts and Adult Mental Health Literature Review: addressing the evidence base from participation in arts and cultural activities.* Durham: University of Durham (CAHHM); 2004.

42 Secker J, Hacking S, Spandler H, *et al. Mental Health, Social Inclusion and Arts.* London: National Social Inclusion Programme; 2007. Available at: www.socialinclusion.org. uk/resources/index.php?subid=71 (accessed 30 July 2008).

43 Cowling J, editor. *For Art's Sake? Society and the arts in the 21st century.* London: ippr; 2004.

44 Arts Council England. *Local Government and the Arts: a vision for partnership.* London: Arts Council England; 2003.

45 Local Government Association. *The Future of Mental Health: a vision for 2015.* London: Sainsbury Centre for Mental Health; 2006.

46 Turner, Senior, op. cit.

47 Ministere de la Culture et de la Communication. *First European Forum on the Arts in Hospitals and Healthcare.* Paris: ADCEP; 2002.

48 CREATE. *Report on the Dublin International Arts and Health Conference.* Dublin: Arts Council Ireland; 2004.

49 Smith T. *A Report on Common Knowledge's Six Hour Coffee Break.* Durham: University of Durham (CAHHM); 2001. p. 3.

50 University of Northumbria. *Tyne and Wear Health Action Zone Evaluation: patterns of engagement and entrenchment.* Newcastle: University of Northumbria; 2001.

51 Department of Health. *Choosing Health: making healthier choices easier* [White Paper]. London: Department of Health, 2004.

52 City of Liverpool. *The Art of Inclusion: Liverpool's creative community.* Liverpool: Liverpool City Council; 2005.

53 Arts Council England, Department of Health. *A Prospectus for Arts and Health.* London: Arts Council England; 2007.

54 Department of Health. *A Report on the Review of the Arts and Health Working Group.* London: Department of Health; 2007.

55 Ibid. p. 3.

56 Arts Council England. *The Arts, Health and Wellbeing.* London: Arts Council England; 2007.

57 Mirza M, editor. *Culture Vultures: is UK arts policy damaging the arts?* London: Policy Exchange; 2006. Available at: www.policyexchange.org.uk (accessed 30 July 2008).

58 Ibid. pp. 105–6.
59 Friedli L, Griffiths S, Tidyman M. The mental health benefits of arts and creativity for African and Caribbean young men. *J Health Promot.* 2002; **1**(3): 32–45.
60 Mental Health Foundation. *Strategies For Living.* London: Mental Health Foundation; 1997. Revised 2000.
61 Mirza, op. cit. p. 103.
62 Vajpayee SAB. Speech at the 58th Session of the UN General Assembly. New York: 25 September 2003. Available at: www.un.org/webcast/ga/58/statements/indieng030925.htm (accessed 30 July 2008).
63 Carey J. *What Good Are The Arts?* London: Faber; 2005. pp. 167–8.
64 Williams R. *Towards 2000.* London: Chatto and Windus; 1983.
65 Watt G. Policies to tackle social exclusion. *BMJ.* 2001; **323**: 175–6.
66 Dissanayake E. *What Is Art For?* Seattle, WA: University of Washington Press; 1988.

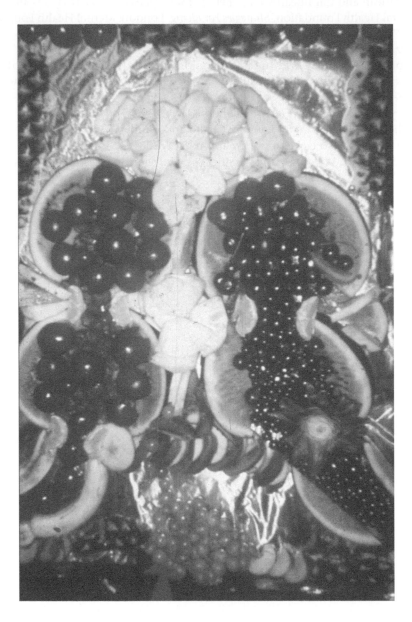

Fruit sculpture illustrating blood flow in the heart.
PHOTO: CENTRE FOR ARTS AND HUMANITIES IN HEALTH AND MEDICINE

# CHAPTER 2

# Finding the crossroads

The major theme of health education is prevention. However since a person's health is inextricably linked to the quality of life, the primary aim of health education and promotion should be to create.

David Seedhouse, *Health: the foundations for achievement*[1]

I have traced the path of arts development in community health in the UK over the last two decades, noting the events that have marked its route and the challenges and obstacles encountered. This chapter looks at the course of thinking in public health that has sought to influence new social and political agendas and at the opportunities this opens for the joint collaboration of the arts, health and education sectors. Recent inquiry into the economics of well-being and how public value is determined also has bearing on locating the crossroads where these sectors can together find a new and meaningful role in community health development.

## THE NEW PUBLIC HEALTH

The emergence of arts in community health in the 1980s coincided with a shift in public health thinking away from the behaviourist approach of health education to a wider context of health promotion that recognised the social determinants of health. In some ways this 'new public health' reconnected with its origins as a civil movement in the nineteenth century, reclaiming the moral crusade of health as a right of citizenship, but it also recognised the interrelationship of individuals and their environment as a key health determinant. John Ashton has defined it as:

> an approach which brings together environmental change and personal preventative measures with appropriate therapeutic interventions. The New

> Public Health goes beyond an understanding of human biology and recognises the importance of health problems which are caused by lifestyles . . . the environment is social and psychological as well as physical.[2]

Creativity has been seen by some key figures in this field, such as Ashton and Seedhouse, as both a means of and an end to expressing health as a quality and not just a biological state. The new public health signalled the framing of a social rather than biomedical model of health in which the creative capacity of individuals and social connectedness are important drivers for achieving community well-being.

The impetus for this change came in 1978 when, under the auspices of the World Health Organization (WHO), leaders in public health from both developed and developing nations met at Alma Ata in the former Soviet Union to frame a declaration that the improved well-being of citizens was to be the millennial goal of global public health. From Alma Ata forward, public health specialists began to think in terms of developing new social norms for health, empowering people toward personal growth and responsibility for their health actions, making increased use of the media for health education, and building alliances and support systems that would enable individuals to make healthy choices.

The prompt for the Alma Ata Declaration's shift in approach had actually come decades earlier. The WHO's 1948 definition of health as 'a state of complete physical, mental and social well-being and not merely the absence of disease or infirmity' had moved it from the hegemony of a biomedical model to a social model.[3] Although flawed in its utopianism, this definition has since become popularised to the point of symbolising a paradigm shift. The WHO definition is commonly understood as describing individuals, but, with regard to the WHO's aspirations in the decades that followed, it may be more correct to see it as applicable to peoples. In this context, 'complete' can be seen not as an absolute term but rather as used in the sense of 'joined together'.

The Alma Ata Declaration[4] led to the WHO's *Health for All* strategy in 1981.[5] Beguiled by the belief in a 'new world economic order', it had a vaulting ambition to achieve an equitable distribution of basic public health resources worldwide by 2000. *Health for All* in turn influenced the Healthy Cities movement, which saw the value of learning and cultural exchange from the experience internationally of cities that signed up to this common programme. Within this context, the strength and nature of local culture was seen as an important indicator of health.[6] It seemed the more local and specific that the interpretation of *Health for All* goals became, the more that cultural activity emerged as a key factor in their realisation. Attention by public health policy-makers to what constitutes a healthy city has been paralleled in the cultural policy sphere by analysis of factors that drive the strategic development of the 'creative city'.[7]

Common to both is a concern to support social inclusion by fostering meaning, identity and a sense of place through cultural engagement.

This is crucial too to the realisation of the WHO definition of health. As the moral philosopher Peter Baelz observed, 'To stress the importance of a vision of a healthy society is to set health in the context of culture and to relate it to human values.'[8] He argues that health education should be about getting people to live towards the future in which connectedness is greater than just self-interest. He cites Michael Wilson and James Mathers, a social psychologist who worked with Wilson at Birmingham in the 1970s, as pioneers in this thinking. He continues, 'Health education is never simply the imparting of information by one who knows to one who does not know. It is a communication of insights, shared exploration of a shared humanity, *a venture of persons in the making*' (my italics).[9] I would suggest that what Baelz is pointing towards here is a form of social capital originating in a quality relationship around the communication of health.

This relationship-based approach to health, coupled with Seedhouse's assertion that health is 'creative potential', has been an important driver in the practice of arts in community health, as I shall explore in the next chapter. Were this approach integrated into the strategic development of the 'creative city', it could impact not only on nurturing healthier communities but also on the local economy. This is why Gateshead's arts in health programme described in the previous chapter was an important element of a local arts development platform that could strengthen the case for major capital investment in Tyneside's new cultural facilities of the BALTIC gallery and the Sage international concert hall. More recently, health has been an important programme theme in European Capital of Culture festivals in Cork in 2005 and Liverpool in 2008.

For the arts to have an effective role in communicating health awareness through social integration, it is important to see that the burgeoning field of arts in community health has not come about solely as a result of the community arts sector making an advocacy pitch to the health sector; it originates just as much in health thinking of the last quarter century, especially in the rise of this new public health movement. A key document in formulating the new public health philosophy was a 1974 report by Canadian health minister Marc Lalonde titled *A New Perspective on the Health of Canadians.*[10] Two years later, when Ottawa hosted the WHO First International Conference on Health Promotion, the principles of health promotion within the new public health movement were set out in a charter.[11] I can see these principles are just as applicable to the practice of arts in community health; namely in the charter's assertions that:

➤ health promotion actively involves the population in the setting of everyday life rather than focusing on people who are at risk for specific conditions and in contact with medical services

➤ health promotion is directed towards action on the causes of ill health

➤ health promotion uses many different approaches which combine to improve health
➤ health promotion depends particularly on public participation
➤ health professionals – especially those in primary healthcare – have an important part to play in nurturing health promotion and enabling it to take place.

The 1986 Ottawa conference also placed emphasis on development skills in order to foster autonomy through education in formal and informal settings.

As it became clear that the *Health for All* strategy was far off achieving its ambitious targets for 2000, it was revised and then renewed in nations with advanced economies in 1998.[12] How the WHO's goal of a global equity in public health might be attained could be viewed differently, however, from divergent cultural perspectives. The problem is succinctly expressed in the Commission for Africa report (2005), which makes an interesting generalisation across the North–South global divide on the connection between social and economic development, well-being and culture:

> What is development for? Many in Western countries see it as being about places like Africa 'catching up' with the developed world. In Africa, by contrast, you will be more likely to be told something to do with well-being, happiness and membership of a community. In the West development is about increasing choice for individuals; in Africa it is more about increasing human dignity within a community.[13]

Focused into the context of health development (and the morbidity and mortality rates in Africa are where the commission report begins), these distinctions seem even more apparent. The title of the 2004 public health White Paper for England, *Choosing Health*,[14] appears superficially to equate individuated healthier lifestyle with sensible consumerism, whereas the Commission for Africa report's subtitle, *Our Common Interest*, makes the collective call for change advocated in 2005's Live 8 campaign.[15] In the perspective of global public health and interdependency, where issues of rights and citizenship are coming to the fore, a vibrant culture may provide a means to link both individuated and collective approaches to improving health status.

In the keynote Leavell Lecture to the World Federation of Public Health Associations conference in April 2004 in Brighton, Ilona Kickbusch argued that global health needs to move out of the charity mode into the realm of rights, citizenship and a global contract, and she underscored action on the globalisation of public health with a principle of social science theory: 'the understanding of health as an end (the right of citizenship) is as important as the utilitarian principle of health as a means.'[16]

What the public health sector has perhaps recognised more palpably than the arts sector is the need for effective joint working between agencies to deliver both the means and end. John Ashton has described public health in the UK as a function rather than a discipline and sees that it requires cross-sector initiatives. In *Public Health and Primary Care: towards a common agenda*,[17] he warns of public health being subsumed within primary care and calls for the development of a model to organise services and plan education and research, but he sets out some caveats for this. He warns against a too-narrow view of health promotion and against the assumptions that activists are normative (i.e. just existing healthcare staff), and that the sum of parts can equal the whole (i.e. without taking on board social exclusion issues). He considers that it is a priority to reconcile conflict between individuated and collective approaches to improving health.

A parallel can be drawn here with arts in health practice; there has often been a too narrow view of the field, with art being required to work within a medical model of services and treatment, and there have been assumptions that the artist alone is the arts in health practitioner rather than the cross-sector relationship that drives the work, that the therapeutic qualities of art activity can deliver benefits without addressing social determinants of health, and that unless a diversity of approaches by arts to health is embraced there could be conflict over the prioritisation of what makes for good practice.

Ashton sees the five key elements for public health research as: positive indicators from qualitative data, a focus on context as well as people, doing things from where people are, true stories, and an assessment of the health-promoting capabilities of communities. This echoes the principles of the Ottawa Charter but turns up the volume on user-led service design. In advocating a grounded theory approach to public health research, Ashton challenges the evidence-led decision-making that has confounded social innovation in public health through adherence to the empiricism that determines clinical governance.

Ashton's caveats have been addressed but not exactly removed by the measures introduced in *Choosing Health* and the 2004 Public Health Act.[18] In his keynote address to the UK Public Health Association Forum in 2005 in Gateshead,[19] Ashton raised the following points in relation to this Act: that there has been a sea change in government thinking from illness to health models; that public health often looks in the wrong place for the health gain and needs to be more lateral in its approach; that the acid test lies in being prepared for future not historical health challenges, e.g. an obesity epidemic; that risk conditions are as important as risk factors, especially where lack of autonomy is a cause of ill health; and that how to die properly is a public health issue. In this bullet-point salvo, Ashton underlined that a change in thinking without a widening of vision will prove ineffective in tackling both the social and moral determinants of public health.

John Ashton and Howard Seymour's book *The New Public Health* draws a distinction between bottom-up health promotion that looks at the big picture in epidemiology and a top-down didactic health education that takes a narrower behavioural-change view. Their book notes 'a real conflict' between the clinical model based on individual transactions and the public health model based on a social contract with entire communities. It calls for social entrepreneurs in public health and acknowledgement of health promotion as professional work but not a profession per se. Sociability is seen as a key requirement, providing a pathway to effective open learning:

> Open learning is a special type of *participation*, and it is a very necessary part of a mass programme. It means providing on a large scale learning environments through which people can *choose* to start at a point which suits their present state of development, knowledge, skills, emotional involvement etc., and then embark on a journey which is under their control and provides them with their own unique experience – an experience which is unique to them and can be catered for within a mass programme. The reason for open learning and the other factors outlined is to encourage people to join a journey of self-discovery. To do this people must be motivated. All the processes outlined are ways of gaining motivation – motivation to change, without having a detailed long-term professional style relationship, without unacceptable cost and loss of control, and with choice and freedom. Fun and enjoyment are also highly motivating and part of this approach. Learning and the motivation to learn are greatly enhanced by making the process one which is attractive and enjoyable. There are two main ways to gain change. One is to change the world and people adapt to fit the new circumstances, and the other is for people to want to – to be motivated to – change and to have the tools and facilities to do it. Both are major aspects of the practice of health promotion. The first relates to political, policy and environmental change, the second to the *populist approach*.[20]

The value structures that inform and the processes that shape this kind of 'open learning' chime with the ethos of arts in community health, though once again Ashton argues for a 'mass programme' of cultural education around health. Participation may not be as generalisable as he suggests. Arts in community health works on a much smaller scale, based on the adaptability of its methods in diverse contexts rather than their strict replicability. State intervention for lifestyle change can be intimidating to the very people it seeks to support. Striking a balance between the two approaches that Ashton outlines would require locally specific and sustained examples of 'open learning' that can measure personal and social change.

## THE PIONEER HEALTH CENTRE

What Ashton terms the 'populist approach' was first articulated at the Pioneer Health Centre at Peckham in South London in the 1930s. This centre was established by pathologist Dr Scott Williamson and medical registrar Dr Innes Pearce. Their main purpose was to undertake an investigation into the nature of positive health and into the nature of the circumstances in which health can be cultivated. The Pioneer Health Centre was later to be seen as a prototype for the healthy living centres.

An account of the Pioneer Health Centre, *Being Me and Also Us* by Alison Stallibrass, a one-time member of the centre, relates that members of the centre did not think of health as a state; rather they thought of it as a way of acting and of relating with an environment. She asserts that the community members' self-esteem and joy in life were increased by the development of their potential capabilities: 'When families get together in an environment that is rich in opportunity for all of them, a force of incalculable power is released. If health is a process of mutual subjective synthesis of organism and environment and of person and group, it is not something that members of the medical profession can give us. They can only remove or alleviate the pathological conditions that prevent us from engaging in the process of health'.[21]

Scott Williamson saw that the challenge of addressing working people's health needs required both realism and imagination, because, as Stallibrass puts it, 'To change the environment of their working lives or their housing was too big an undertaking for a small group and too long-term, but to change their leisure-time environment was a possibility'.[22] Observation of that leisure time was the basis of what Williamson termed a long-term 'experimental station in human biology' at the Pioneer Health Centre. From its modest non-building-based beginnings in 1926, it raised funds through subscriptions to realise a groundbreaking architectural design and use of a purpose-built community leisure facility in the 1930s, until the war and some decline in usage with the coming of the NHS forced it into closure in 1951. The building was constructed predominantly in glass around a central swimming pool, with interior glazed walls enabling users to observe a range of activities. These activities included drama, dance and crafts, taking place simultaneously with encouragement for inter-generational leisure pursuits. The centre's minimalist design by Sir Owen Williams was praised by the Bauhaus' founder Walter Gropius as a fine example of the public health architecture that flourished in the inter-war years, exempli-fied in lidos and sanatoria, that aimed to enhance public buildings with the perceived virtues of sunlight, fresh air and open vistas.[23]

A generation later, the lessons of the Peckham Experiment began to be picked up again in the public health arena in a more formative way. Alex Scott-Samuel's review[24] of the experiment's achievements notes that what particularly distinguished the centre was its focus on activities that combined spontaneity with responsibility in an environment that fostered social support and integration. He speculates that any future projects modelled on Peckham will be family-oriented and multi-generational, and that they might be found either in an existing situation that offers opportunities for growth or be created anew in favourable circumstances. One can see the legacy of Peckham in healthy living centres such as Bromley-by-Bow and Looking Well, which will be described in later chapters.

## HEALTH AS A SOCIAL IDEA

The WHO's *Health for All* strategy in 1981 eventually instigated a sea change in public health thinking, even though the millennium false-dawned with the WHO's ambitious goals having failed to translate into global political action on health inequalities. The new agenda for public health, based on the European Region's response to the WHO *Health for All* strategy,[25] only began to be implemented in the UK 25 years later. The new paradigm for public health was interrupted in the Thatcher era by a focus on health as an exchange model based on a service economy, virtually ignoring the Black Report on social inequalities in health, which was also published in 1981.[26]

That year, Ilona Kickbusch published a seminal paper on the (then) innovative 'lifestyle' concept of health behaviour change. Kickbusch begins her paper by declaring, 'Health is a social idea. Virtually every programme seeking to protect, maintain or improve health has social and behavioural aspects.'[27] Her paper refers to several basic orientations being required: new images of health, innovative educational approaches, lay participation, a multidisciplinary approach, new strategies on various levels, and social and environmental factors that influence health decisions. I note in particular that she says 'a social model of health sees self-reliance as an expression of human dignity and development',[28] bringing a contemporary reinterpretation of Samuel Smiles' *Self-Help* (1859) to public health thinking.

This self-reliance tenet has been reinforced by the growing interest from public health policy makers in a 'health assets model'. This contends that historically health promotion has worked on a deficit model that is focused on the problems and needs of communities to be addressed through health resources. An asset model, on the other hand, looks at communities' capability and capacity to identify problems and activate their own solutions, so building their resilience and self-esteem. A WHO European Office report[29] argues that salutogenic (or health-generating) factors that generate health awareness through social cohesion and personal meaning are as important as pathogenic (or sickness-generating) processes, particularly as risk factors account for only 40–50% of early mortality. Identified health assets in a community include wisdom, creativity, talent and enthusiasm, and these reveal cultural and values-based potentiality. Tapping into these assets 'may require new training and reorientation of existing social welfare and economic delivery and development systems', and the report concludes that 'community cohesion may be a very significant value-based asset with cultural determinants.'[30]

In the contemporary public health arena, the development of health assets in a community is seen to require the nurturing of health literacy, which is defined by the WHO as 'the cognitive and social skills of individuals to gain access to, understand and use information in ways that can promote good health'.[31] One summary document informing UK health policy on prevention and patient involvement states that 'there is a need to develop a broader based investigation that goes beyond medically determined studies to include sociological research. This is vital in order to look specifically at differences between groups in decision-making capability and preferences'.[32] The Alliance for Health and the Future, however, sees that broader investigation of health literacy must include 'a critical empowerment strategy' in which 'health messages and solutions must be placed within settings relevant to their target audiences and encompass both a social and health dimension'.[33] For effective health messaging to inspire public confidence and motivation to change, it has to be about more than information and access to services, so an assets-based model of health needs to look at producing a wider gamut of activity and engagement. There is a danger that health literacy can become circumscribed to the relationship between users and services, rather than an improved ability in the population to 'read' the health implications of lifestyle, social connections and environment.

A framework that could practically assist a health-assets approach in the public health sector's work with communities was set out in the 2006 government White Paper *Strong and Prosperous Communities*,[34] which proposed arrangements for local authorities to lead on health and well-being issues in local communities. It aimed to shift the pattern of healthcare provision to prevention, with particular attention to complex issues of social exclusion. It encouraged movement at local level towards joined-up actions through connected care plans and the development of patient-led controlled budgets that respond to patients' expressed needs and wants (particularly in mental health), and local councils are now empowered to make joint appointments with health services for directors of public health and other senior NHS appointments.

The *Prosperous Communities* White Paper had an accompanying strategy for third-sector commissioning. This has paved the way for a culture change in commissioning, providing opportunities for the voluntary sector to bid to run programmes and services, while recognising that some organisations will be small (many have income of less than £50000 per annum) and not have capacity for observing the big bid protocols. This could be a significant strategic change that could assist in getting arts projects into community care partnerships, based on local area agreements forged between local authorities, primary care trusts

(PCTs) and other partners. The initiative began in 2007, and marked a shift in key local authority services away from direct delivery to a commissioning role. It placed emphasis on the voluntary sector's ability to assist needs assessment and capacity-building in communities, and it advocates more joint workforce development.[35] Further government support for this shift came in summer 2008 with the publication of the Empowerment White Paper,[36] which set out how the untapped talent of communities can be unleashed to create improvements to public services, local accountability and opportunities for enterprise.

Health and well-being have already featured as a key aim of most local authorities' cultural plans, and in 2003 the Local Government Association (LGA) and Arts Council England jointly affirmed an aim to integrate arts and health into local strategic partnerships.[37] I believe this is now fertile ground for arts in community health, and as I described in Chapter 1, most of my own experience of developing work in this field has been done under a local authority aegis. Health trusts are so target-driven that arts practice within them can find itself so compartmentalised and instrumentalised to address health priorities that there is little breathing space to explore what makes for the effective public engagement of creativity with health. In local authorities, on the other hand, the attention has been more broadly on quality of life and environment and on public satisfaction with service provision.

The 2006 White Paper, in empowering local authorities to share control of the public health function, requires them to set improvement targets related to desired national outcomes on health and well-being. Strategies to deliver on these targets must remain sensitive to local culture and circumstances, or the inherent advantage of having local authorities as a commissioning nexus for services relevant to local population needs may be lost. Measures in the 2008 White Paper, however, could help safeguard against this happening. It is more than health issues and priorities; it is about ways of living, identity, meaning and place – and these are essential factors in the development of arts in community health.

## AN ECONOMICS OF WELL-BEING

New thinking in public health has been informed by an evolving theory of the economics of well-being, in which participation in social activities is seen as a powerful determinant of health and happiness. Robert Bellah and William Sullivan relate how the post-war vision of John Maynard Keynes and William Beveridge for the economy and welfare state were founded on a moral belief in cultivating 'goodness' in society and not the material ends in themselves. This, they say, sets out a 'third way' in politics between market and state domination: 'It is time we turned our attention to developing the *symbolic resources* [my italics] which can enable citizens to interpret their concerns in ways that connect to the vision of human betterment with equity and solidarity that is the moral heart of progressive politics'.[38] The 'third way' expounds a theory of progressivism based on cooperative enquiry, shared values and participation. It sees modern communities as involving multiple overlapping memberships, and it sees the goods of a positive welfare society as being autonomy, health, education, well-being and initiative. In arts in community health, these 'goods' are delivered in a broad range of social outcomes arising from engagement in creative activities, often with 'symbolic resources' shaped by the creation of new traditions in a community's social calendar.

The progressivism that Bellah and Sullivan describe has entered the health arena in efforts to motivate the public to participate in the design and delivery of their healthcare services. There is a role here for arts in assisting health-needs assessments, in visualising what makes for a healthy community and in communicating the social value that underpins healthcare in the process of consultation itself. Creating a climate of positive regard is crucial if the move to user-led services is to succeed. Liz Kendall and Lisa Harker[39] forecast how social services will be run in combination with other agencies in 2020, and they argue that it requires a citizenship model rather than a consumer model of care to take people out of 'dependency' culture. It is foreseen that a realignment of professional boundaries will be required, as will the creation of new hybrid professions, and that joint working arrangements between local authorities and NHS services must not be dominated by the NHS. Under a citizenship agenda, preventative healthcare is about fostering responsibility both in individuals and in communities and then providing holistic yet targeted services to vulnerable groups. But such a pragmatic agenda could become a rationale for 'downsizing' services, so it needs to be underpinned by both a clear strategy for the public's participation in the design of health services and by the humane principles of an economics of well-being.

A focus on addressing the needs of vulnerable groups has placed mental health at the forefront of a shift to patient-centred care in the community, and this focus points to the need for change in the economics of health. The World Health Organization predicts that by 2020 mental ill health will be the second greatest cause of debilitating illness in developed nations (after heart disease),[40] and the Mental Health Foundation already estimates that one in five children will develop a mental health problem by the time they reach adulthood.[41] In 2006 the London School of Economics (LSE) published *The Depression Report*,[42] highlighting that one in three families at some point will have a member requiring treatment for depression, while only 2% of the NHS budget is spent on this service. The LSE called for 10 000 more therapists to be trained as a proven successful alternative to medication, and it has done some persuasive maths to justify the cost.

The intervention of more therapists should not be the only approach to a growing epidemic of distress. The LGA's partnership strategy paper *The Future of Mental Health: a vision for 2015* recognises a broad approach is required that draws on what all the public services in its remit have to offer.[43] It supports the move for mental health service clients to have more say in their treatment plans through personally devolved care budgets. This is an opportune time for promoting arts in mental health directly to service clients and the wider public and for building pathways between arts and art therapies in institutional care and arts initiatives in the community that integrate mental health service users. Arts can have a role in both prevention of mental ill health and post-discharge recuperation, as the LGA paper acknowledges: 'Key to promoting mentally healthy communities are initiatives to build confidence and self-esteem, for example, by enabling affordable access to sport and leisure, cultural, artistic and other activities.'[44]

In local authorities there has been a growth of subsidised referral schemes from health services to cultural activities. Stockport Council's 'Arts on Prescription', for example, was introduced in the mid-1990s and has been widely replicated elsewhere.[45] For the most part, however, these have been small-scale initiatives and often not sustained beyond a trial period. The 'prescription' tag has tended to circumscribe the activity to a discrete intervention with individual patients rather than to shape a broad alignment within communities of health and cultural services. The 'affordable access' that the LGA advocates should not be limited to determining concessionary rates for health service clients but must consider what constitutes an economics of well-being for whole communities.

To convey the bigger picture, the New Economics Foundation has produced *A Well-being Manifesto for a Flourishing Society*.[46] It sees three interlinked factors for well-being that are not addressed in economic indicators: personal satisfaction with one's life, personal development and social well-being. It is claimed that a 20% increase in income only produces a short-term increase in well-being. Well-being is accounted for by genes (50%), by circumstances (only 10%) and by outlook and activities, including arts and sports (40%). It is in the latter area that a difference can be made, particularly if user satisfaction becomes the key indicator in public service delivery. The manifesto concludes with the same concern voiced by public health in that 'our present system has it the wrong way round: the centre tends to specify the means rather than the ends',[47] thereby hampering on-the-ground initiatives that are locally tailored to tackle these areas for action. The manifesto's preoccupation with creating meaningful work for people, however, makes it a bit snobby on the effects of TV and mass culture, and it disregards the financial considerations that may determine what sort of work people choose to do.

The New Economics Foundation's 'well-being manifesto' calls for the creation of a set of national well-being accounts.[48] It points out that the government's 2005 sustainable development strategy[49] was committed to exploring well-being indicators, and the 2006 European Social Survey produced a module on well-being from a questionnaire designed by the New Economics Foundation.[50] One result of that questionnaire suggests that the actual nature of an activity is less important to well-being than the fact that it affords interaction with other people and opportunities for personal development. This should caution against making exaggerated claims for the efficacy of arts or other interventions in isolation, and it indicates that attribution of the benefit to the participants is far more complex. While arts in community health could have a useful role alongside a range of potential cultural interventions delivered through museums, libraries, sports, green spaces etc., there is a question as to whether it is superficially any more effective than, say, bingo. While a post-modernist take on culture and well-being might suggest 'anything goes' if it achieves social integration, a qualitative difference must lie in the depth of meaning that can evolve through the activity. François Matarasso has compared the instrumental and intrinsic values of the arts and observed that:

> Many of the benefits of being involved in community arts are also associated with helping on an environmental project or being in a parent teacher association: they are the benefits of participation rather than of the arts. The essential reason why the arts are so important to society is not the socio-economic outcomes they share with other activities, important as those are, but the human and cultural outcomes which are wholly distinctive to them – questions of identity, meaning and values, and all the otherwise inexpressible thoughts and feelings that we are.[51]

The 'economics of well-being' has evolved a rationale as to why social engagement through culture can be an influential variable in people's perceived life satisfaction, but has so far neglected consideration of the respective merits of, and the extent of effects arising from, different kinds of activity – probably because this is so complex to measure and is affected by the meaning and value that each individual attaches to them. As Matarasso suggests, however, socioeconomic outcomes are subservient to fuzzier human responses whose impact in the public realm is persuasive by consensus rather than by being empirically demonstrable.

Establishing qualitative differences in the impact on health of interventions across the cultural sector requires attention first to how they are pitched and delivered. A broad-based approach to identifying and promoting the effects that culture can have on both personal and social well-being could usefully align itself with the growing interest in the public health field in social marketing. The National Consumer Council's report on social marketing[52] offers a rationale for campaign approaches in public health, defining social marketing as 'the systematic application of marketing concepts and techniques, to achieve specific behavioural goals, to improve health and reduce inequalities'. It says health promotion has to begin with people's value systems and that 'establishing "behavioural goals" requires going beyond the traditional focus on "behaviour change" to recognise the dynamic nature of behaviour within a whole population.'[53] Social marketing combined with the kind of open learning that Ashton describes could be a potent means of delivering mass-messaging that also touches and motivates people at a personal level. This is why interventions that bring together arts, health and education sectors could be at the forefront of this.

To sum up: the 'new public health' has opened the way for cultural development to have a role in addressing health inequalities and in improving the relationship between health services and the public. It promotes an assets model of community health in which the creation of social value can impact on wellbeing rather than just focusing narrowly on individual behaviour change. Health literacy needs to be conceptualised and promoted in this wider context, supported at ground level by the lead role that local authorities have been given in developing local strategic partnerships for health and social care. An economics of well-being requires qualitative assessment of cultural impacts, but with effective social marketing a nexus of arts, health and education sectors to develop community health could be achieved. I now want to look at the importance of the 'feel-good factor' in producing individual and social well-being and how engagement with the arts contributes to that.

## STATUS, INEQUALITY AND SOCIAL CAPITAL

Research suggests behaviour change depends significantly on a feel-good factor. Arts in health project reports frequently refer to the improved feeling of self-worth of participants. Increased self-esteem is cited, for example, as a key indicator in Matarasso's *Use or Ornament?* study of the social impact of the arts.[54]

In Australia, VicHealth's 1999 report *Art for Health*[55] gathered information on self-esteem impacts arising from arts involvement through questionnaires completed by 90 arts organisations. VicHealth reported that 91% stated that their work contributed to health improvement in the local area by developing people's self esteem, and 82% stated that participants' confidence increased as a result of participation.

The claim that participatory arts improve self-esteem needs to toughen up, however. Self-esteem is not necessarily always a good thing; some of us could do with less of it. A more pertinent watchword may be dignity. What has always impressed me about successful dance projects with elderly people, for example, has been the inherent dignity of both the process and the participants' responses. Dignity might be measurable too in that we all have an instinctive understanding of when our own has been violated. As Richard Horton, editor of the *Lancet* observes, 'Injuries to individual and collective dignity may represent a hitherto unrecognised pathogenic force with a destructive capacity towards physical, mental and social well-being at least equal to that of viruses and bacteria.'[56] The ability of the arts to help counter this would be worth demonstrating, particularly as the related factors of improved confidence and well-being are commonly cited as benefits by participants in arts in health projects.

Self-esteem is also a powerful factor in the social gradient of health, as evidenced in the work of Sir Michael Marmot on status. In *Status Syndrome*, Marmot makes a persuasive case that social status is the biggest single determinant of health, even when allowing for variation in economic conditions and lifestyle habits:

> All societies have rankings because individuals are unequal in a variety of ways; but not all societies have the same gradients in health. What matters is the degree to which inequalities in ranking lead to inequalities in capabilities ... the lower in the hierarchy you are the less likely it is that you will have full control over life and opportunities for full social participation. Autonomy and full social participation are so important for health that their lack leads to deterioration in health.[57]

This thinking, which is informed by 30 years of solid international research, could be an important basis on which to develop evaluation of arts in health projects in areas of high social and economic deprivation. The research shows that people and places both matter for health. More deprivation in an area means worse health. Lower social position also means worse health – and the two can interact. Related issues are home and community safety, access to amenities and social capital. In a newspaper feature (*The Guardian*, 16 February 2005), Marmot states:

> We found that trust, tolerance and sense of attachment to the neighbourhood were strongly connected to health. These links were independent of the physical infrastructure. Interestingly the links of social cohesion to health were stronger among women than men. The likely explanation was that for women involved in childcare, the social cohesion of the neighbourhood is of vital importance.[58]

Marmot therefore argues that social cohesion should be a central focus of policy and planning and that ghettoisation of low-income/low-status groups should be remedied. The oft-cited hierarchical 'pyramid of human needs', devised by Maslow,[59] places esteem and dignity in the second highest position below self-realisation, but Marmot shows that these are much more fundamental needs.

Underlying these issues of self-esteem and status, and what the arts can do to improve them, is the relationship between dignity and health, which Horton describes as a pathogenic condition. This relationship also should inform development considerations in global public health. Horton goes on to say that:

> People may be poor in material terms without that having any direct bearing on their dignity. Likewise compromised dignity, unlike income poverty, cannot be resolved by economic aid alone. Aid can only go so far in helping to create the conditions for human dignity.[60]

Horton believes a measurable scale for assessing maintenance of dignity in relation to overall health ought to be possible, and he refers to the work of epidemiologist Jonathan Mann in this regard. Further research is required on this.

Richard Wilkinson's fascinating book *The Impact of Inequality: how to make sick societies healthier*[61] reveals a clear correlation between economic and health inequalities and explores the effect this has on perceptions of social status, levels of crime and social disaffection. Initially he takes a dim view of culture, seeing it as a marker of inequality in a modern class system: 'The aesthetics of those at the bottom of society serves to define the "bad" taste that provides the ground against which "good" taste is socially constituted.'[62] He considers psychosocial factors to be important because they go to the heart of a person's subjective experience of the quality of life. So feelings are key to health, especially the shame of low status. He argues that to understand class we need to think more about our evolution from apes than our ideological debt to Marx. He says:

> If the health effects are the effects of low social status, then we can see how their impact could occasionally be offset by a sense of community, by a sense of identity . . . the most important psychosocial risk factors are the most important sources of stress.[63]

A central argument is that the relationship between income inequality and health is mediated through the quality of social relations. Higher income inequality leads to higher health inequality, deterioration of social capital and escalation of violence – and he asserts that there is global evidence of this.

Wilkinson inspirationally brings together epidemiology, psychology, economics and evolution theory, and he lays down a political challenge. He puts forward evidence that health is better where the status of women is better, and he shows that wider social capital is built on 'bridging' rather than 'bonding' forms, e.g. extended family. Looking at evolution, he says that from two million years ago brain size grew as language and culture developed and this happened in order to deal with social relations. An egalitarian society of foragers predated the hierarchical society of agriculture based on tackling scarcity. Our social life now has varying degrees of the two social systems. Much depends on how our childhood experience demonstrates the kind of social structure we may live in as adults. He gives an interesting account of stress hormones and their effects and notes a recent study that showed via an MRI scanner that social exclusion is a physical pain. When finally acknowledging the importance of cultural interactions on health, he says:

> Also crucial to friendship and mutuality are our powers to empathize and identify with others. In addition to their direct effects, these abilities are also essential to the capacity for imitative learning, which is the foundation of a cultural way of life.[64]

This is also a basic tenet of art education and emotional intelligence, and, as expounded in the work of US art commentator Ellen Dissanayake,[65] it motivates the biological necessity of art-making in almost all societies.

Wilkinson has emphasised the health benefits arising from a more cohesive society. She argues that the quality of the social life of a community is one of the most powerful determinants of health and that this is related to the degree of income inequality. The sociologist Ray Pahl agrees, seeing that the quality of our social relationship in micro-social worlds is coming to be regarded as having a vital role in maintaining and achieving better health. Pahl also points out that income inequality is not the whole story, and that it is feelings of self-esteem and of being valued, coupled with close personal relations and wider social networks, that have bearing on health. Pahl, however, challenges Wilkinson's idea of social support existing within each social strata, whether it be in the workplace or in the family, and how these systems of social support are important in health maintenance and morbidity prospects.[66] What Pahl seems particularly concerned with is that so far Wilkinson and the social capital theorists have not adequately defined and described what these systems of social support are. In this respect, it would be worth looking at how informal systems of social support are evolved through cultural programmes, specifically in arts in health and related fields of disability arts, arts for elderly and children's art projects that involve parents. A dialogue here between sociologists, epidemiologists and arts workers could prove mutually helpful and establish a basis for multidisciplinary research.

Robert Putnam, an American political scientist, puts the negative effects of asocial acquisitive behaviour squarely down to the erosion of social capital. In his book *Bowling Alone*,[67] he reported that Americans now tend to bowl alone rather than in leagues. This is a symbol of a disappearing 'togetherness' as measured by a decline in all sorts of communal behaviour within social capital. He has quantified this term, and his measurements show that communities with lots of social capital tend to have higher health status, better schools, less crime and so on. Researchers at the London School of Economics have used some of this thinking to analyse whether areas in Britain with greater social capital (as defined by Putnam) have higher levels of health.[68] They found that predominately they do. It has also been shown that engagement with wider social spheres improves physical and mental health and promotes recovery.[69] This requires that social networks and opportunities – for employment, housing, leisure and friendship – become the central concern of mental health service providers, rather than being considered a secondary gain from efficiently implemented care programmes.

In *Bowling Alone*, Putnam introduces his chapter on health and happiness with the declaration that 'Of all the domains in which I have traced the consequences of social capital, in none is the importance of social connectedness so well established as in the case of health and well-being.'[70] He cites research demonstrating that happiness is best predicted by the breadth and depth of one's social connections, and the extent of a person's civil connections rival marriage and affluence as predictors of life happiness. This in turn has direct bearing on health, because apparently the more integrated we are with the community the less likely we are to experience colds, heart attacks, strokes, cancer, depression and premature death of all sorts.

The term 'social capital' was originally coined by James Coleman in 1988 to emphasise the preconditions for social life, as distinct from the material conditions of social existence (physical capital) and the attributes of individual social actors (human capital).[71] Unfortunately, through over-use 'social capital' has become a mix of all these, often idealised and unsubstantiated, and it gets cited as both a precondition and result of successful health intervention in community contexts. Some key flaws have been pointed out in social capital theory. McQueen-Thompson and Ziguras[72] note that the term 'social capital' has been used almost synonymously with 'community' and 'social networks' in social health projects literature. It has become a catch-all phrase, loosely defined without recognition that it is a very contested term in sociology, and it is sometimes used to express the summative outcome of different indicators of benefit. There is also a conundrum in social capital theory as to whether it has demonstrable externalities beyond the value to the individual, making it a communal attribute.[73]

Social capital theory has now found currency internationally in different societies, cultures and healthcare systems, but it is too often used just to beef up discussion about the value of participation in cultural life. For example, in setting out an approach to local arts development in New Zealand in her book *Cultural Well-being and Cultural Capital*,[74] Penny Eames seems to conflate social capital and cultural capital. Referring to Bourdieu's *The Forms of Capital*,[75] she argues that social capital comes from the core of cultural capital, not vice versa, and that we should look at the asset values of behaviours and how they impact on social and economic well-being. Her assertion that behaviours are what we look for in culture, and the networks are the social capital, reveals perhaps how a precondition and a result get confused, and she later makes a rather discomforting suggestion that cultural development can be a way of 'rebranding' a community to exploit its assets, overlooking complex issues of autonomy and self-determination. Nevertheless, she is addressing a robust policy framework and refers throughout to the New Zealand Local Government Act 2002, which is based on the 'four pillars' of sustainable development: social, economic, environmental and cultural well-being. (Interestingly, the policy accommodates a Maori-influenced view of prosperity to include prosperity of spirit, family and harmony.)

Eames defines cultures as having three phases: emergent, mature and rigid. They reach their apogee in mature cultures that manifest the kind of adaptive inclusiveness that Richard Florida sees as characteristic of creative cities.[76] Eames' book is let down, however, by a finale 'practical section' that is little more than a summary of what should go into framing a local cultural strategy, and she fails to deliver on her intention to show how cultural capital can be measured. One factor in the confusion over social and cultural capital is that theorists have given their attention to identifying outcomes rather than describing process. Process is vital to understanding how the arts work and engage with people.

The community arts sector needs to figure more largely in social capital research. Marmot and Wilkinson do not adequately explain the structure and processes of social support that can mitigate the effects of health inequalities, perhaps because looking at the cultural aspects of this is not in their domain. Likewise, Putnam focuses more on the level and degree of participation in civil society rather than how and why participatory activities are developed. In the rush to defining outcomes, the statistical formulae he produces for quantifying social capital can be baffling. For example, in his essay *The Social Context of Wellbeing*, he suggests that you can calculate from his data the overall effect of age on subjective well-being by 'multiplying the coefficient in the variable in question in the health equation by the health coefficient in the wellbeing equation and adding this indirect effect to the direct effect of the same variable in the well-being equation', and he then concludes, 'In other words, living in a high-trust community seems to improve health.'[77] Ironically, it is hard to place one's trust in this kind of 'science' of social capital.

A better understanding, I think, of the social psychology that goes into building trust and reciprocity in communities is expressed in a book that predates social capital theory, Lewis Hyde's seminal work on arts and the gift economy, *The Gift*.[78] Hyde contrasts the sterile exchanges of commodity culture with the ability of an artwork or totem to bind a community through an evolving tradition of reciprocal generosity. Making artwork as a social gift is at the heart of thinking and practice in community arts. A gift is not a commodity at all, in the sense that its value is perceived wholly in the transmission rather than the accumulation of a good. What matters is the sentiment and ceremony of the process. As Hyde describes it:

> When a gift passes, it becomes the binder of many wills. What gathers in it is not only the sentiment of generosity but the affirmation of individual goodwill, making of those separate parts a *spiritus mundi*, a unanimous heart, a band whose wills are focused through the lens of the gift. Thus the gift becomes an agent of social cohesion, and this again leads to the feeling that its passage increases its worth, for in social life at least, the whole is greater than the sum of its parts.'[79]

This seems to me to connect with that earlier description by Baelz of meaningful health information being 'a venture of persons in the making';[80] and interestingly, Richard Sennet has defined the criteria for social inclusion as mutual exchange, ritual and witness to others.[81] Hyde emphasises the importance of a process of emotional transaction through creative participation that makes for genuine empowerment rather than a balance sheet deduction of how much social or cultural capital a community may possess. Indeed, by their works ye shall know them.

## NEW APPROACHES TO HEALTH EDUCATION – AND MISSED OPPORTUNITIES?

In the context of how a 'gift economy' can creatively bind individuals into communities, arts in community health could make an important contribution to providing practical examples of the 'fully engaged scenario' recommended in the Wanless Report to the UK Treasury, *Securing Our Future Health*.[82] The Treasury responded to the Wanless Report by commissioning further research from Wanless' team into this scenario, which suggests that in the long term, by 2020, health spending will have levelled out as a consequence of more direct engagement by the population with self-care approaches (coupled with improvements in medical and information technologies). The Royal College of General Practitioners' summary report on the Wanless Report states that patients do not visit GPs when they have sustained access to more informal support networks (GP visits reduced by up to 46%), that patients do not use mainstream services if they have been trained to take care of some of their long-standing problems (hospitalisations reduced by up to 50%) and that patients require less medication if they have knowledge or the confidence to manage their conditions in other ways (outpatient visits reduced by 17%). The RCGP summary also notes:

> Initial Department of Health estimates suggest that investing around £200 per person with a long-term condition results in savings and quantifiable benefits

of double that amount, as a result of fewer GP visits, decreases in hospital admissions and visits, and a reduction in the number of prescriptions and the drugs bill. Taking possible costs of special measures to manage risks into account, the net benefits are estimated at £150 per person.[83]

While there are clearly implications here for proper clinical governance of patients whose condition is acute, there is much potential for arts in health work to assist people at risk, long-term patients or people post-discharge, and thereby assess comparable reductions in care spend.

Although the Wanless Report heralded an opportunity for public health to reclaim a social agenda as set out in the 2004 White Paper *Choosing Health*,[84] what has tended to become sidelined is the importance of the 'deep sociality' that Wilkinson describes as a key determinant of health and happiness. That White Paper did, however, seem reflective of public opinion gleaned from a lengthy national consultation, and it acknowledged that previous approaches to public health had been too top-down. Its strategy for democratising public health was further reinforced in 2008 by Lord Darzi's 'next stage review' of the NHS, titled *High Quality Care For All* which called for every primary care trust to commission comprehensive well-being and prevention services, in partnership with local authorities, with the services personalised to meet the needs of their local population.[85] Key issues in both *Choosing Health* and *High Quality Care For All* are informed choice, personalisation and working together – and priorities are smoking, obesity, exercise, alcohol, sexual health and mental health. *Choosing Health* pioneered a plan to create 2500 children's centres, 3000 community matrons and 400 sports academies. There was, surprisingly, no reference to the arts in the White Paper, despite Arts Council England's own submission to the consultative process.

*Choosing Health* promised that successful community-based models for improving health could be more confident of sustained support, although this has been somewhat contradicted in how its improvement measures have been designed and implemented. It saw the importance of identifying grassroots health champions, who signpost people to local services and work with them on personal health plans. The overall aim was for the NHS to become a 'health improvement and prevention service'. The LGA would have a key role in delivery, in partnership with primary care trusts. Arrangements were outlined for mental health patients to propose self-care plans, and there were more efforts to redress inequalities in ethnic minorities' access to mental health services. The report concluded that there was huge public support to create an irreversible momentum for change. It called for an innovations fund to test new models of working and to focus on capacity-building in the workforce by sharing modular training with other sectors.

*Choosing Health* emphasised that its key aim was 'personalisation of support to make healthy choices', and it made a commitment to establishing a Health Trainers initiative. Expressions of interest from designated 'spearhead' primary care trusts and their potential partners were invited, and it was mandatory that a scheme on which it would be possible to model a Health Trainers initiative should already be running. This resulted in 78 partnerships (comprising primary care trusts, local authorities, academic institutions etc., and geographically covering nearly half the NHS) for inclusion in an 'early adopter phase' implemented in 2005–06. In a written statement to the House of Commons in July 2005, the (then) public health minister, Caroline Flint, described the health trainer as 'a new kind of personal support in the public health work force', recruited on the basis of their 'people skills' and local knowledge, not necessarily previous health service experience'[86] – a rather ironic turnaround from Aneurin Bevan's assertion in a 1949 radio broadcast that 'The NHS will never be a substitute for the good neighbour.'[87] The Health Trainers initiative aimed to become England-wide by 2007.

From the outset, the trainers were envisaged as 'lifestyle coaches' providing one-to-one advice and support, constraining the wish in some 'spearhead' partnerships to take a more community-based approach based on a healthy living network model. Health trainers are placed in a range of settings, reaching into communities that professionals find hard to reach, and are offered a qualifications framework for career development. They also have a covert role gathering intelligence from communities. The focus has been on trainers as paraprofessionals, unlike the informal lay health workers advocated a generation earlier by Michael Wilson. Wilson felt it was important that these informal workers' inherent strengths should not be hindered by a professional label:

> Every community has its key people to whom others turn in a crisis. They are the carriers of a society's culture and therefore the actual builders or destroyers of health. They are key people in any attempt to change a society's attitudes or values in relation to health, illness, life and death.[88]

On the child development and education front, *Choosing Health* took a 'whole school' approach to health, with children at risk to receive personal health guides and with the aim for all schools to achieve a healthy school standard by 2009. The Health Promoting Schools Award scheme is a partnership between primary care trusts and education services, and it is led by healthy schools workers in the cities and sub-regional areas. The Healthy Schools Standard (HSS) progresses incrementally to a level-three accreditation (integrated programme with constant monitoring and review), with special attention given to schools in deprived areas. Local flexibility, and in some cases a track record in using arts, makes HSS an important ally in developing schools-based arts in health work that addresses public health priorities. Schools are supported, guided and evaluated in their work by an HSS project officer. The aim is to achieve a whole-school culture shift in key health issues relevant to the local community. It does this by introducing small changes in policy and behaviour that will be sustained over the long-term to bring improved health and attainment for pupils and staff. HSS routinely evaluates interventions in the short and medium term to assess attitudinal change in audiences/participants. This could offer a baseline for quantitative evaluation of arts impact on child health.

The HSS initiative looks assured until at least 2010. It has been further strengthened by guidance from the National Institute for Health and Clinical Excellence on promoting children's social and emotional well-being,[89] which recommends HSS should be developed alongside the Social and Emotional Aspects of Learning (SEAL) programme[90] and 'related community-based initiatives'. The SEAL programme addresses the 'personal, social and health education' module in the school curriculum, which was introduced in 2001, and it provides the opportunity for health to be treated not just as a subject but as part of the ethos and culture of a school. This converges with what was advocated in the 1999 government review of creativity in education, *All Our Futures*, which stated that 'creative and cultural education are not subjects in the curriculum but general functions of education.'[91]

*All Our Futures* concluded that:

> Teaching for creativity aims to encourage: autonomy over the ideas being offered; authenticity from decisions based on one's own judgment; openness to new ideas, methods and approaches; respect for each other and for the emerging ideas; and fulfilment in the creative relationship. Above all, there has to be a relationship of trust. This can encourage a sense of responsibility for learning, leading to self-directed learning involving goal-setting and planning, and the capacity to monitor, assess and manage oneself.[92]

This parallels the principles of behavioural change in public health promotion and offers a viable basis for developing health education in schools. This connection, however, has yet to be made practically through arts in education. Although I title this chapter 'Finding the crossroads', it is clear that sometimes paths are traversed in the dark and opportunities are missed. *All Our Futures* helped give birth in 2002 to Creative Partnerships, Arts Council England's massive arts in education programme that was targeted into over one thousand schools in 36 areas of high social and economic deprivation. It was jointly funded by the Department for Culture, Media and Sport and the Department for Education and Skills. There were, however, surprisingly few examples of this programme engaging with health issues and local health services.

## SOCIAL VALUE AND THE ARTS FUNDING SYSTEM

At the same time as Creative Partnerships rolled out nationally, two consecutive publications from the national office of Arts Council England (ACE) set a context for project delivery in arts in health. The first of these, *Ambitions for the Arts*,[93] committed ACE to establishing an effective partnership with the Department of Health and looking locally at partnerships with key organisations already engaging in arts in health. It says:

> Without compromising our main purpose – the arts – we will make the most of growth by establishing effective partnerships with a range of national, regional and local organisations. Nationally, these include government departments for health, education, trade & industry, and the Home Office as well as agencies such as the Youth Justice Board and national broadcasters. Regionally and locally, these include regional development agencies, regional government offices, local strategic partnerships, regeneration agencies and, of course, local authorities.

A measure of success for *Ambitions for the Arts* is 'more teachers, health professionals, probation officers, youth workers, social workers and carers reporting the value of the arts in their work.'[94] A follow-up publication, *Ambitions into Action*,[95] declares that as the result of shared vision, 'the arts are playing a powerful role in realising the ambitions of those in health, education, crime reduction, civil renewal, regeneration and other issues that touch the lives of people throughout the country.'[96] The problem was that, apart from Creative Partnerships, this 'shared vision' had not led to much research-informed strategic development that would place these alliances in national programmes to share workforce development, practice and evaluation. It did, however, signify a shift in ACE's policy and research interests away from the focus on the economic importance of the arts during the Thatcher era, exemplified in the Myerscough Report,[97] to an investigation of the social impact of the arts that began with Matarasso's study *Use or Ornament?*[98]

Despite an understandable reluctance to compromise on its main purpose, the arts, the validity of ACE's bold statements in *Ambitions for the Arts* as to the transforming nature of the arts requires better evidence of an alignment of cultural and social values in its funding policies. Indeed, ACE's chief executive, Peter Hewitt, went further in calling for investigations that would attempt to show that it is possible to have a better understanding of the circumstances, factors and characteristics that go towards delivering special impact in arts and culture.[99] This would require a complex but overdue inquiry into what constitutes quality in arts practice and into public perceptions of how the subsidised arts impact on society and individuals.

A Demos 'think tank' report, *Capturing Cultural Value*,[100] gave a timely and interesting analysis of how the social value agenda could revitalise the relationship between funders, funded and public, exploring the tension between instrumental approaches and intrinsic 'art for art's sake' approaches to identifying cultural value and social outcomes. It calls for a language that can 'make explicit the range of values addressed in the funding process to encompass a much broader range of cultural non-monetised value . . . the argument is that an essential part of the process of creating value flows directly from the actions and existence of the provider organisation itself as well as from the experience and satisfaction of the citizen.'[101] This tests whether the users agree with the organisers. Getting meaningful public support for a community arts project, however, takes time and considerable organisational commitment to develop. The report suggests adapting perspectives from anthropology, environmentalism and 'intangible asset' accounting. In assessing funding applications, there would have to be a plurality of 'languages' in order to discuss different kinds of cultural intervention – and this process may require even more evaluation and feedback. I believe the process of assessing applications needs rather to be simplified. Despite these complications, the Demos report offers a more holistic framework to assess and support arts interventions, and it empowers the funded organisations to state their mission and review their actions against their own values. The word 'health' as a core value occurs throughout this report.

Similar arguments were to be found in a US report titled *Gifts of the Muse: reframing the debate about the benefits of the arts*, which was commissioned by the Wallace Foundation.[102] This US-speak document needs some 'translation', but the gist is that the arts need to reinstate their intrinsic as well as instrumental benefits and distinguish between private and public benefits. The report sees studies of health and social benefits as being limited so far in methodology and data. It notes a weakness in the attribution of benefits (because health benefits could be due to other effective causes than arts) and considers that the most important instrumental benefits require sustained involvement in the arts. It argues that intrinsic benefits are not solely private but include the creation of social bonds and communal meanings. The trouble with promoting 'intrinsic benefits', however, is that we go back to 'art for art's sake' arguments and still focus on the individual experience more than the communal.

In 2005 ACE and the Arts and Humanities Research Council jointly commissioned the Centre for Cultural Policy Studies at the University of Warwick to undertake new research into the social impact of the arts. An interim summary paper on this research deplores how public debate on the value of arts has come to be 'dominated by what might best be termed the cult of the measurable', and how it has become inseparable from funding issues.[103] The paper argues that the tension between intrinsic and instrumental arguments is a sterile dichotomy. It then sets out a taxonomy of claims for the arts in a historical context under three headings: a negative tradition (from Plato onwards), a positive tradition (from Aristotle and the humanists) and the autonomy tradition (from aestheticism) that rejects instrumental approaches. It concludes that policy debate has been detached from historical traditions that could help to provide debate on the value of the arts with the language some say is missing. I think it could be argued that it is equally detached from the 'user's voice'. The taxonomy of claims for the arts that this paper presents is focused on products, not processes. Participants' testimony about the effect on them of the processes of arts engagement would provide useful information on what is valued in the arts. Historical background is useful, but a policy debate still has to be in a contemporary context.

In 2006, as a lead-in to its national arts debate, ACE held a series of regional consultative meetings in an attempt to get a cross-section of public opinion on how the arts are regarded and valued.[104] Those meetings concluded that amongst the most commonly perceived benefits of the arts were that they create a sense of identity for individuals and communities and they assist improvement of mental and physical health. Surprisingly perhaps, other social, educational, political and economic benefits were deemed less significant. Contention over public spending on arts in healthcare was focused on commissioned works of public art, which have been the mainstay of arts in hospitals. Recognition, however, of a link between participation in the arts and the promotion of individual and communal well-being was broadly accepted.

There appeared to be little concern with drawing distinctions between intrinsic and social benefits, provided three criteria for an artwork are met: an original creative idea, the skill and effort that goes into executing that idea and transforming it into an end product, and the achievement of a response from an audience. So what constitutes aesthetic quality seems for most people to be refreshingly simple, and this is felt, at least intuitively, to be causative of personal improvement and social value. Engagement with the arts is viewed by the public as a matter of personal choice and taste, but it is seen as engagement, not just passive consumption. This augurs well for participatory arts practice that is sensitive to social inclusiveness being regarded as a common good.

Within the parameters of the national arts debate, it could be argued that arts in community health should come to the forefront of the arts in health movement, as it demonstrates an engagement that touches lives and communities. Arts in community health could also help mediate public response to conceptual art within healthcare environments by establishing the validity of art for communicating health and supporting service delivery. Arts in community health might lay claim to being a kind of conceptual art itself; it is just that the concepts are evolved through community participation.

The national arts debate had a lengthy period of open consultation following on from the regional meetings, and this debate involved ACE staff, members of the public, artists, arts managers, local authorities and other key stakeholders in several hundred interviews, discussion groups and deliberative events. There were also over 1200 contributions to the open consultation.

A concluding report[105] describes the arts debate as ACE's first public value inquiry. It was further confirmed that the well-worn internal debate over intrinsic versus instrumental values of arts participation seemed irrelevant to most people. The social dimension of engaging with the arts was seen as important, and this was readily associated with friendship and diversity. The report claims participants in the debate perceived that the public value of the arts lies in three domains: building capacity for living, enriching the experience of life and providing 'powerful applications' in contexts beyond the arts experience itself, where, for example, 'at an individual level [the arts] offer an outlet for emotions and a means of expressing what might otherwise be difficult to say. As such they can contribute to overall health and emotional wellbeing.'[106] The emotional response to an artwork is thus also held up as an arbiter of its quality. Public value is identified in people's aspiration for state funding to focus on achieving some tangible social outcomes that benefit not just those who take part in the funded activity but the wider community as well, though some in the arts field might worry that social engineering is being encouraged entry by rear-door access. It was claimed that social engagement through the arts leading to empowerment was crucial. The summary concludes that the ultimate end of public funding for the arts should be the creation of public value in terms of the three domains referred to earlier, and that the twin priorities of artistic excellence and public engagement become critical means of achieving this overarching ambition. The summary is light on statistical findings, however, offering instead a rather specious comparison: the ACE costs each UK household 39p per week and the NHS costs around £80 per week.

Coincidentally perhaps, the Department for Culture, Media and Sport moved swiftly to reinstate the pre-eminence of artistic innovation with the McMaster Report,[107] which was instigated by a new secretary of state, James Purnell MP. The McMaster Report's conclusion – that a greater sense is required of what excellence is within public discourse on culture – is somewhat at variance with ACE's impression from the arts debate of the sophistication of public opinion about the arts. Sir Brian McMaster's report uses the word 'culture' throughout as a vague substitute for 'the arts', seeing it as a commodity that is presented to the public as an offer it cannot refuse. The 'cultural offer' emerged from the margins of the 2007 arts debate to become a catchphrase as government encouraged schools to engage pupils in up to five hours a week of cultural activities and a pilot scheme for this was initiated the following year. Questions around whose culture and what it comprises were left unaddressed by McMaster. Consequently, the ideological tensions in the arts field affecting the practice of arts in health that I described in Chapter 1 seem as unresolved as ever.

McMaster settles on innovation as the marker of excellence, overlooking that the arts are also steeped in their traditions, but he at least affirms a humanist base to his review by defining an excellent cultural experience as one that 'goes to the root of living'. It could be argued that a person's state of health might also be found at that root. As I have tried to show in this chapter by drawing in thinking from public health, economics, education and the arts, the potency of a relationship between the cultural experience and one's state of health is primed for exploration. For that relationship to flourish, what needs to be better understood at this juncture are the characteristics of practice that inform the process of arts development in community health; in short, defining the attractions inherent in this work. This is the subject of the next chapter.

## REFERENCES

1 Seedhouse D. *Health: the foundations for achievement*. Chichester: Wiley and Sons; 1980. 2nd ed. 2001. p. 121.
2 Ashton J, Seymour H. *The New Public Health*. Milton Keynes: Open University; 1988. p. 21.
3 World Health Organization. *Preamble to the Constitution of the World Health Organization*. New York: Official Records of the World Health Organization 2; 1948. p. 100.
4 World Health Organization. *Declaration of Alma Ata*. Proceedings of the International Conference on Primary Health Care, 6–12 September 1978. Alma Ata, USSR. Available at: www.who.int/hpr/NPH/docs/declaration_almaata.pdf (accessed 30 July 2008).
5 World Health Organization. *Strategy for Health for All by the Year 2000*. New York: WHO; 1981.
6 Hancock T. The evolution, impact and significance of the Healthy Cities/Communities movement. *J Public Health Policy*. 1993; **14**(1): 5–18.
7 Landry C. *The Creative City: a toolkit for urban innovators*. London: Earthscan; 2000.
8 Baelz PR. Philosophy of health education. In: Sutherland I, editor. *Health Education: perspectives and choices*. London: Allen and Unwin; 1979. p. 29.
9 Baelz, op. cit. p. 32.
10 Lalonde M. *A New Perspective on the Health of Canadians*. Ottawa: Ministry of Supply and Services; 1981. Available at: www.hc-sc.gc.ca/hcs-sss/com/fed/lalonde-eng.php (accessed 30 July 2008).
11 World Health Organization. *The Ottawa Charter for Health Promotion*. New York: World Health Organization; 1986. Available at: www.who.int/healthpromotion/conferences/previous/ottawa/en/ (accessed 30 July 2008).
12 World Health Organization. *Health21: the health for all policy framework for the WHO European Region*. Copenhagen: WHO; 1998. Available at: www.euro.who.int/document/health21/wa540ga199heeng.pdf (accessed 30 July 2008).
13 Commission for Africa. *Our Common Interest: an argument*. London: Penguin; 2005. p. 28.
14 Department of Health. *Choosing Health: making healthier choices easier* [White Paper]. London: Department of Health; 2004.

15  Wikipedia. *Live 8*. www.en.wikipedia.org/wiki/Live_8 (accessed 12 August 2008).

16  Kickbusch I. The end of public health as we know it: constructing global health in the 21st century. *Proceedings of the World Federation of Public Health Associations Conference, 19–22 April 2004*. Washington, DC; World Federation of Public Health Associations; 2004. p. 9. Available at: www.wfpha.org/Archives/Transcript%20of%20Leavell %20Lecture1.pdf (accessed 31 July 2008).

17  Ashton J. Public health and primary care: towards a common agenda. *Public Health.* 1990; **104**: 387–98.

18  Department of Health, *Choosing Health*, op. cit.

19  United Kingdom Public Health Association Forum. *Renewing Public Health: renaissance and responsibility.* London: United Kingdom Public Health Association; 2005.

20  Ashton, Seymour, op. cit. p. 87.

21  Stallibrass A. *Being Me and Also Us: lessons from the Peckham experiment.* Edinburgh: Scottish Academic Press; 1989. p. 254.

22  Ibid. p. 20.

23  Worpole K. *Here Comes the Sun: architecture in public space in twentieth century European culture.* London: Reaktion; 2000.

24  Scott-Samuel A. *Total Participation, Total Health.* Edinburgh: Scottish Academic Press; 1990.

25  World Health Organization. *Health21: the health for all policy framework for the WHO European Region*, op. cit.

26  Department of Health. *Social Inequalities in Health: report of a research working group* [the Black Report]. London: Department of Health; 1981.

27  Kickbusch I. Involvement in Health: a social concept of health education. *Int J Health Educ.* 1981; **24**(4): 3–15.

28  Ibid. p. 8.

29  Harrison D, Kasapi E, Levin L, *et al. Assets for Health and Development: developing a conceptual framework.* Venice: European Office for Investment in Health and Development; 2004.

30  Ibid. p. 9.

31  World Health Organization. *Health Promotion Glossary.* Geneva: WHO; 1998. p. 10.

32  Sihota S, Lennard L. *Health Literacy.* London: National Consumer Council; 2004. p. 7.

33  Kickbusch I, Wait S, Maag D. *Navigating Health: the role of health literacy.* London: International Longevity Centre UK; 2007. p. 18.

34  Department of Communities and Local Government. *Strong and Prosperous Communities: the local government White Paper.* London: Stationery Office; 2006.

35  Department of Health. *No Excuses. Embrace Partnership Now. Step Towards Change: report of the Third Sector Commissioning Task Force.* London: Department of Health; 2006.

36  Department of Communities and Local Government. *Communities in Control: Real People, Real Power* [The Empowerment White Paper]. London: Stationery Office; 2008.

37  Arts Council England. *Local Government and the Arts: a vision for partnership.* London: Arts Council England; 2003.

38  Bellah RN, Sullivan WM. Cultural resources for a progressive alternative. In: Tam H, editor. *Progressive Politics in the Global Age.* Cambridge: Polity; 2001. p. 22.

39 Kendall L, Harker L. *From Welfare to Well-being: the future of social care.* London: ippr; 2002.

40 Murray CJL, Lopes AD. Alternative projections of mortality and disability by cause 1990–2020: global burden of disease study. *Lancet.* 1997; **349**: 1498–1504.

41 Mental Health Foundation. *The Big Picture.* London: Mental Health Foundation; 2000.

42 Centre for Economic Performance. *The Depression Report: a new deal for depression and anxiety disorders.* London: London School of Economics; 2006.

43 Local Government Association. *The Future of Mental Health: a vision for 2015.* London: Sainsbury Centre for Mental Health; 2006.

44 Ibid. p. 16.

45 Huxley PJ. *Arts on Prescription.* Stockport, UK: Stockport NHS Trust; 1997.

46 Shah H, Marks N. *A Well-being Manifesto for a Flourishing Society.* London: New Economics Foundation; 2004.

47 Ibid. p. 8.

48 Northwest Culture Observatory. *Culture and Health.* Preston: Culture Northwest; 2006.

49 UK Government. *Securing the Future: a strategy for sustainable development.* Stationery Office; 2005.

50 New Economics Foundation. *Personal and Social Well-being Module for the European Social Survey, Round 3.* Available at: www.cambridgewellbeing.org/Files/Well-being-Module_Jun06.pdf (accessed 31 July 2008).

51 Matarasso F. *The Weight of Poetry: the unique challenges of evaluating the arts.* 2002. p. 6. Available at: http://homepage.mac.com/matarasso/ (accessed 31 July 2008).

52 National Consumer Council. *It's Our Health: realising the potential of effective social marketing.* London: National Consumer Council; 2006.

53 Ibid. p. 39.

54 Matarasso F. *Use or Ornament? The social impact of the arts.* Stroud: Comedia; 1997.

55 VicHealth. *Art for Health.* Melbourne: VicHealth; 1999.

56 Horton R, editor. *Second Opinion: doctors, diseases and decisions in modern medicine.* London: Granta; 2003. pp. 491–512. p. 505.

57 Marmot M. *Status Syndrome: how your social standing directly affects your health and life expectancy.* London: Bloomsbury; 2004. p. 248.

58 Marmot M. For richer, for poorer. *Guardian.* 16 February 2005. Available at: www.guardian.co.uk/society/2005/feb/16/socialcare.health (accessed 1 August 2008).

59 Maslow AH. A theory of human motivation. *Psychol Rev.* 1943; **50**: 370–96.

60 Horton, op. cit. p. 509.

61 Wilkinson RG. *The Impact of Inequality: how to make sick societies healthier.* Abingdon: Routledge; 2005.

62 Ibid. p. 176.

63 Ibid. p. 89.

64 Ibid. p. 259.

65 Dissanayake E. *Homo Aestheticus: where art comes from and why.* Seattle: University of Washington Press; 1992.

66 Pahl R. Some sceptical comments on the relationship between social support and well-being. *Leis Stud.* 2003; **22**: 1–12.

67 Putnam R. *Bowling Alone: the collapse and revival of American community.* New York: Simon and Schuster; 2000.

68 Campbell C, Wood R, Kelly M. *Social Capital and Health*. London: Health Education Authority; 1999.
69 Sayce L, Morris D. *Outsiders Coming In: achieving social inclusion for people with mental health problems*. London: MIND; 1999.
70 Putnam, *Bowling Alone*, op. cit. p. 326.
71 Coleman JS. Social capital in the creation of human capital. *Am J Sociol*. 1988; 94: 95–120.
72 McQueen-Thomson D, Ziguras C. *Promoting Mental Health and Wellbeing: a review of literature focussing on community arts practice*. Melbourne: VicHealth; 2002.
73 Putnam R. Social Capital: measurement and consequences. *Proceedings of OECD workshop*; 19 March 2000; Paris. Available at: www.oecd.org/dataoecd/25/6/1825848.pdf (accessed 1 August 2008).
74 Eames P. *Cultural Well-being and Cultural Capital*. Wellington, NZ: PE Consultancy; 2006.
75 Bourdieu P. The Forms of Capital. In: Halsey A, Lauder H, Brown P, *et al.*, editors. *Education: culture, economy and society*. Oxford: Oxford University Press; 1997.
76 Florida R. *The Rise of the Creative Class*. New York: Basic Books; 2002.
77 Helliwell JF, Putnam R. The social context of wellbeing. In: Huppert FA, Baylis N, Keverne B, editors. *Science of Well-Being*. Oxford: Oxford University Press; 2005. p. 453.
78 Hyde L. *The Gift: how the creative spirit transforms the world*. New York: Routledge; 1979. Republished Edinburgh: Canongate; 2006.
79 Ibid. p. 36.
80 Baelz, op. cit. p. 32.
81 Sennet R. How work destroys social inclusion. *New Statesman*. 31 May 1999: 25–7.
82 UK Treasury. *Securing Our Future Health: taking a long-term view* [the Wanless Report]. London: HM Treasury; 2001.
83 Royal College of General Practitioners. *Summary Paper: Wanless report 'Securing our Future Health'*. London: RCGP; January 2002. p. 9.
84 Department of Health, *Choosing Health*, op. cit.
85 Darzi A. *High Quality Care For All*. London: Department of Health; 2008. Available at: www.dh.gov.uk/en/Publicationsandstatistics/Publications/PublicationsPolicyAndGuidance/DH_085825 (accessed 3 January 2009).
86 Secretary of State for Health. *Notice of Written Ministerial Statement on Health Trainers*. London: House of Commons; 20 July 2005.
87 BBC Archive. *Bevan, Rt Hon Minister of Health: one year after its introduction, the founder speaks on the Health Service*. Available at: www.bbc.co.uk/archive/nhs/5150.shtml (accessed 1 August 2008).
88 Wilson M. *Health is for People*. London: Darton, Longman and Todd; 1975. p. 105.
89 National Institute for Health and Clinical Excellence. *Promoting Children's Social and Emotional Well-being*. London: NICE; 2008.
90 Department for Education and Skills. *Excellence and Enjoyment: social and emotional aspects of learning*. London: Department for Education and Skills; 2005.
91 Rogers R, editor. *All Our Futures: a summary*. London: National Campaign for the Arts; 2000. p. 5.
92 Ibid. p. 6.
93 Arts Council England. *Ambitions for the Arts*. London: Arts Council England; 2003.

94 Ibid. p. 14.

95 Arts Council England *Ambitions into Action*. London: Arts Council England; 2004.

96 Ibid.

97 Myerscough J. *The Economic Importance of the Arts in Britain*. London: Policy Studies Institute; 1988.

98 Matarasso, *Use or Ornament?*, op cit.

99 Hewitt P. The value of evidence . . . and the evidence of value. In: Cowling J, editor. *For Art's Sake: society and the arts in the 21st century*. London: ippr; 2004.

100 Holden J. *Capturing Cultural Value: how culture has become a tool of government policy*. London: Demos; 2004.

101 Ibid. p. 44.

102 McCarthy KF, Ondaatje EH, Zakaras L, *et al*. *Gifts of the Muse: reframing the debate about the benefits of the arts*. Santa Monica: Rand Corporation; 2004.

103 Belfiore E, Bennett O. *Rethinking the Social Impact of the Arts*. Warwick: University of Warwick; 2006.

104 Central Office of Information. *The Arts Debate: regional consultation meetings*. London: Central Office of Information; 2007.

105 Bunting C. *Public Value and the Arts in England: discussion and conclusions of the arts debate*. London: Arts Council England; 2007.

106 Ibid. p. 14.

107 McMaster B. *Supporting Excellence in the Arts*. London: Department for Culture, Media and Sport; 2008.

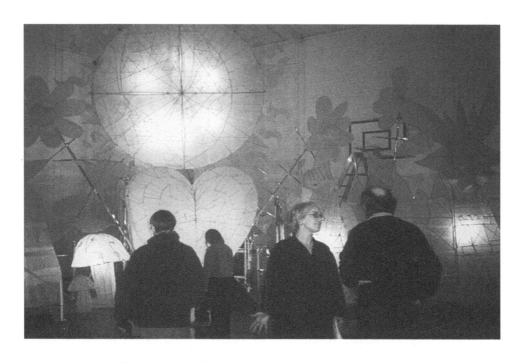

The 'congenial space'. PHOTO: CENTRE FOR ARTS AND
HUMANITIES IN HEALTH AND MEDICINE

# CHAPTER 3

# The characteristics of practice

Not one grand construction, but many small ground works

The Common Knowledge motto

This chapter aims to identify the factors that can make for effective practice in arts in community health and link them to the ethos that underpins the work. It then sets out some common features that establish the identity and purpose of the work in a wide range of community settings.

In considering the characteristics of arts in community health, I do not wish to divorce this work from the rest of the field in which it operates. I see this activity as a distinct strand of arts in health practice, having its own developmental framework and intellectual base. There is still much commonality, however, with approaches to arts in healthcare settings. In both of these practice areas, the therapeutic effects are often embedded in the process and delivery of the art-making, and outcomes are sought as a resonance of this. It is in this respect that hospital arts, art therapies and arts in community health could develop an interesting exchange of research and practice. Therein I believe it might still be possible to evolve a unifying theory of arts in health, which, to have effective influence on policy-makers, is probably needed. Whether the work is located in a hospital entrance, primary care clinic, hospice or sink estate, there is frequently a common purpose to enhance the physical and social environment with arts that provide positive messaging in support of health improvement. A common concern of arts programmes in both hospitals and community settings is to help provide orientation and connection through a supportive sense of place. In the public health arena, there has been growing interest in Aaron Antonovsky's theory of 'salutogenesis',[1] which identifies the origin of health in the human quest for coherence and a harmonious environment,[2] and this could have application across the whole arts in health field.

What distinguishes the pioneering nature of arts in community health is that it is a learning process for all involved, and it is from a multi-sector dialogue that the characteristics of its practice can be best determined. As practitioners themselves may acknowledge, however, some adverse aspects of practice need to be improved or eradicated. There have been lessons learned from both successes and failures; these lessons have informed the impetus in recent years to scale up arts in community health and establish programmes that engage with workforce development in the health sector as well as with service delivery. Increasingly, the work is not just focused on local projects in isolation but seeks to nurture relationships between organisations, their services and the public. A focus on the development of human accord is a defining characteristic of the work, enabling it to be extraordinarily ambitious despite a low resource base.

Different funding regimes for projects are significant in explaining the range and diversity of arts in community health, as the funding sources for the work inevitably have an effect on determining what kinds of approach and thematic content will flourish. Funding must also be a factor in why projects and the organisations delivering them have substantially expanded across many contexts for health and social care in recent years. Audit information on the nature and extent of practice in arts in community health in the UK, and how it is funded, is patchy. I referred in Chapter 1 to a questionnaire survey of arts in community health projects carried out by the Health Education Authority in 1998, which produced 90 responses from organisations and is the only national overview to date of the field. This survey, which was published by the Health Development Agency in 2000,[3] indicated that financial support from health service budgets was sporadic and sparse. Local audits produced under the aegis of Arts Council England's (ACE) regional offices are selective of projects across the arts in health field, are pitched for advocacy purposes and do not estimate the overall level of activity and spend. However, in its publication *The Arts, Health and Wellbeing*,[4] ACE's national office states that between 2003 and 2007 the regional offices had together funded 441 arts in health projects with a total value of awards of £6.5 million, an average award being just under £15 000.

Arts-sector funding is only a small part of the overall picture, however. Largely due to the tenacity and resourcefulness of practitioners, there have been many funding sources for arts in community health, and there is barely a statutory or non-statutory funding regime in the UK that has not been accessed somehow and somewhere to support the work. It would therefore seem superfluous to urge arts in health practitioners to address a cross-cutting agenda; the funding mix suggests they are already doing that.

Because of this diversity of practice, it has proved difficult to source information that might provide a coherent overview of the arts in health field and how it is funded, though one can get glimpses of parts of it on occasion. For example, in 2005–07 Anglia Ruskin University and the University of Central Lancashire carried out research into arts and mental health that was jointly commissioned by the Department of Health and the Department for Culture, Media and Sport. The first phase of this research was an audit of practice, which identified around 200 such projects in the UK. From questionnaire returns, it was determined that in a sample of 100 projects there were around 4000 participants, with 16% of these drawn from ethnic groups that mental health services categorise as normally 'difficult to reach'. The annual operational budget per 100 projects is broadly estimated at £4 million plus £3 million in kind, much of which is provided in health service staff, facilities and volunteer input. Fifty-four per cent of projects have been active for five years or more, suggesting that sustainability is a strong feature of the work. Forty-eight per cent of the projects sampled were located in community settings and 38% in mental healthcare settings. Forty-five per cent of projects integrate mental health clients with the wider community, with service users helping to run activity in 57% of projects, suggesting that social inclusion and skills development are important drivers of the work. Twenty-five per cent of projects attempt evaluation of their work.[5]

While this survey information and that of the Health Education Authority's study[6] (*see* Chapter 1) suggest some characteristics of practice, they lack firsthand observation and a discursive framework for practitioners to reflect on their work. Observational studies based on action research methods are crucial to understanding how the field has evolved and what its value systems are based on.

## DEFINING CHARACTERISTICS OF ARTS IN COMMUNITY HEALTH

In 2003 the Centre for Arts and Humanities in Health and Medicine (CAHHM) published *Arts, Health and Community*,[7] which was an in-depth observational study of five arts in community health projects in England. The projects were the Happy Hearts Lanterns in Gateshead, Looking Well Healthy Living Centre in North Yorkshire, South Tyneside Arts Studio for mental health referrals in South Shields, the arts programme at the Bromley by Bow Centre in London's East End, and the West End Health Resource Centre in Newcastle. The projects selected for this study, which was funded by the King's Fund and the Nuffield Trust, were chosen on the basis that they had a commonality of approach, while each also retained certain unique features. The first two projects will be considered more closely in the case examples in Chapter 7. The South Tyneside Arts Studio is a model example for several similar initiatives in North East England, and the last two projects were regarded by the Department of Health as prototype healthy living centres on the launch of that initiative in 2000.

On the structure of these five arts in community health projects, the study concluded that:

➤ arts in community health projects are firmly located in the non-profit-making, voluntary third sector in the sense that they value their autonomy from the state and they engage in innovatory and critical work

➤ fiercely independent, the arts in community health projects stay separate and work with statutory agencies, sometimes in partnership, sometimes crossing statutory/voluntary lines, but they may sometimes take on statutory responsibilities, some of them being funded for doing so

➤ flat, responsive and non-hierarchical organisational structures serve to maintain commitment on the part of all workers, volunteers and users

➤ small is beautiful, and as projects grow bigger so inevitably do their organisational structures and procedures, and adjusting to growth while retaining the guiding ethos of a project has become a major issue

➤ there is a belief that art is for everyone, and if barriers between professionals, workers, volunteers and users are crossed while maintaining boundaries, it may enhance the commitment of all to the project and to each other

➤ the arts in health space must be a safe, calm place to look out for each other with trust, positive regard and respect.

The key points on ways of working in arts in community health projects, as observed in the study, were:

➤ the work of community-based arts in health projects could be said to revive the notion of care in the community

➤ a significant relationship emerged between art, food and alternative therapies – which together affect people's sense of health and well-being

➤ the use of bartering and recognition of mutuality of space, wherein a project trades its resources (say space) to attract other much-needed resources (say artists), were central to both the ethos and economy of projects

➤ voluntary work and voluntary contributions are valued, while at the same time attention is paid to resourcing activities properly and paying salaries at appropriate rates

➤ personal contacts and personal invitations (as opposed to referrals and self-referrals) to activities increase take-up of those activities

➤ the importance is stressed of making immediate response to those articulating needs or offering resources

➤ knowing that everyone can do something is important in any project, but particularly in those based in the community

➤ arts in community health projects have acted as a catalyst for arts and health development in geographical areas other than their own and in other agencies.

To give substance to these observations, a summary of one of the five projects follows in the next section, highlighting how its arts programme served as a catalyst to a wider social regeneration remit.

## BROMLEY BY BOW CENTRE, LONDON

The centre began 25 years ago as a very small project when a new vicar joined the local church. The numbers in the congregation were very low; most people in the local community were, and are, Muslim. The vicar, Rev. Andrew Mawson, had come from working in a leading drugs-prevention project in another part of London – that project had also been developed by a local minister. The drugs-prevention project's entrepreneurial, risk-taking experience shaped the approaches the vicar was to take in Bromley-by-Bow. It is in one of the poorest local authority areas in England, having some of the most disadvantaged and socially excluded communities. Unemployment and crime rates are high. People living in the area experience poor levels of health. Rev. Mawson spent the first two years talking with local community members, generating ideas for projects that might be developed and would be valued. More importantly, he got to know people living locally who could make such developments happen.

The church initiated projects through attracting small sums of money from a variety of sources. The first major project converted part of the premises of the church into a nursery. A carpentry shop was also developed, turning pews into woodwork benches. Artists were then encouraged to use the centre free of charge and, in return, to work for the local community. More projects developed organically: local women and disabled people took up gardening; the disability gardening group then needed pots and used the pottery in the centre to make them; a local artist wanted to join the pottery group and sold her kiln to the group. An important principle emerged: respond immediately. The centre's approach to all people, including those living locally, is 'What can you do for us?' rather than 'How can we help you?' The focus is not on needs – after all, needs change – rather it is on knowing that everybody can do something.

Having started incrementally with minimal financial resources, the Bromley by Bow Centre pitched its position as a community resource in a poor borough adjacent to the City of London to attract funding from a range of public and private sources. In time it set up an office and staff team concerned specifically with fundraising, monitoring and evaluation. Even so, like all voluntary-sector organisations, it has continued to experience problems with funding.

The centre developed a commitment to look at health in an integrated way and work towards the development of a high-quality health clinic providing health and social care. A local GP practice, including health visitors and district nurses, combined with urban regeneration initiatives to offer an integrated programme of arts, health, education, environment and enterprise. The clinic was opened in 1998, and was a nationally recognised prototype for a healthy living centre.

Arts activity had been important from the start in the Bromley by Bow Centre, but when the centre became a healthy living centre, the development of a specific arts in health programme involving the team of health professionals seemed the obvious step. A portfolio has been kept for each project, including a record of everything that has been done, together with commentary from participants. Some of these projects are summarised here to give a flavour of the centre's cultural programme, which links arts, health and education.

➤ *Operative arts with health professionals* – In the reception area of the health centre, an artist sets up a stall once a week creating designs for posters, health information leaflets etc. GPs, district nurses and health visitors from within the Bromley by Bow Centre and from other surgeries and health trusts are encouraged to join in, as relaxation from their clinical work. It provides them with opportunities to do artwork for their personal enjoyment and use, say to display in their surgeries, and to contribute to the creation of health promotion materials.

➤ *The Airways Project asthma and singing group* – This group, the responsibility of a GP, was established for children with asthma (four to 13-year-olds) in consultation with the asthma nurse. Led by an African woman singer, it engaged children in drama and singing. About six children attended each session, with some of their parents joining in. They were personally invited to the group through local community contacts and GPs, and local health centres referred children. A record book is kept of the sessions, in which children, individually and collectively, write, draw or paint how they feel. Illustrations are made to symbolise the songs, and the group recorded some of the songs on tape. The worker adds her own comments on each session.

➤ *Young @ Art* – This group of older people, many of them formerly housebound, meets once a week in the reception area of the centre. It was set up to run alongside the leg ulcer clinic in order to encourage take-up of the services of that clinic and to make waiting to see the nurse more pleasurable, and in these ways it has been effective. As they come and go to the clinic, people engage in a broad range of arts activities. Complementary therapies such as aromatherapy and massage are also available.

➤ *New Beginnings* – This group, with a crèche, is for mothers with newborn babies. It provides opportunities for them to get together, share experiences and problems and create things for their own homes, e.g. ceramics, silk paintings and pottery mobiles.

➤ *Hand and foot printing* – Each week, running alongside the child clinic, an artist has been making handprints and footprints of children in the reception area. The purpose here is to build developmental charts to measure child development and to compare growth over time and comparative growth amongst children.

➤ *The toy library and book box* – This literacy and arts project runs alongside the baby clinic in the reception area of the centre and has an outreach service to support families with preschool children in their own homes. The literacy work includes many different languages, including Bengali, Somali and English. Storytellers and guest readers visit the toy library, as do singers – all from other parts of the centre.

➤ *Portrait painting* – Alongside the baby clinic, and while the toy library and book box are open, an artist sketches and paints watercolour portraits of babies in the reception area for two hours at the request of the parent, usually the mother. The word has got around; there is no need for referrals, and sometimes mothers come to the centre especially for a portrait to be done. The artist engages in conversation with the mother – usually about the child, his or her features and his or her development since the last portrait was completed. One mother has had about 10 portraits done of her three children as they have grown up. It provides an opportunity for the mother to appreciate her child in a different way. Some of the portraits have been printed and, in a frame together, are on the wall. Mothers chat together, pointing out which is theirs and how the children have changed since their portraits were done. Children come and chat to the artist whom they know.

➤ *Food and Art* – This has involved the food co-op and the community café. Volunteers and students are working on food and art projects, considering ways in which to present food artistically, thus making it more appetising.

What is remarkable about the Bromley by Bow Centre is that small-scale activities such as these consistently provide pathways into further education, voluntary service, employment and small enterprise. As the centre has structured itself to tackle local problems on a broad front, it has developed an effective network of relationships across the statutory and voluntary sectors. It has always made the most of its prime asset, its participants. These small arts in health activities need to be seen in the context of larger support services that are run through the centre, which are listed here.

➤ *Enterprise* – The enterprise team at the Bromley by Bow Centre is responsible for helping centre participants set up new business ventures and for nurturing these. Training is offered in organisation skills, book-keeping and marketing, but most importantly, networking and social support is provided, with the long-term aim for people to be self-reliant in their enterprises. Successful enterprises include: a greeting card business developed by two young women, the growing and weaving of willow products, a Bengali drama group that presents plays each year and on special occasions such as weddings, and a Bengali food and catering service. Other businesses such as the café operate within the centre complex, with the centre effectively offering an internal market.

➤ *Education and training* – Linked with enterprise, arts activities and health are experiential education and training programmes. Participants, who are also volunteers, are registered on accredited programmes leading to educational qualifications.

➤ *Community care* – Bromley by Bow Centre, in partnership with the local authority social services department, provides a community care programme for people with physical and mental disabilities. Some people attend all of the sessions, others only some of them. One of the artists acts as a tutor for the community care group. The group does painting, pottery, silk-screening, exercise and gardening. Local volunteers help the community care participants on a one-to-one basis, and they themselves are accredited for this work through a course.

➤ *The Families Project* – This project's purpose is to support parents through activities in the centre and in their own homes. While it is structured, people may attend on a casual basis. One of its main activities is PACT (parents and children together), which is also seen as part of the arts and health programme. This is open to any parents and their children, and parents are referred to it by GPs and the local authority social services department. The Families Project also has a commitment to the centre nursery. It supports parents in their applications for funded nursery places and acts as their advocate. In partnership with the health development team, the Families Project is responsible for the provision of the toy library and book box (*see* above).

➤ *Community links and inter-organisational relationships* – As Bromley by Bow Centre is a community in itself, the main inter-organisational links tend to be between different parts of the centre. The creative director of Bromley by Bow Centre, who also has responsibility for the enterprise team, described the Centre thus:

> The model is one of concentric circles. At the heart is the huge capacity in the centre for social activity. Individual lives orbit around this shaped by two forces: one which gravitates them towards the centre and another, through the enterprise team, that pulses them round. In this concentric circle of individuals, groups of individuals begin to think of ways of making money from what they have been doing as a social activity in the centre. Rotating around the outside of the circles in the outer orbit are businesses that have been launched and continue. People could become self-employed and leave the area but the aim of the Centre is to encourage them to stay in this community and in touch with the Centre. It works because we're all networking, talking with each other, talking with individual people.[8]

In a positive way, this is going round in circles, drawing participants into the central ethos of the organisation as a socialising facility in order to connect them to the wider orbits of education and enterprise. There can inevitably be some complications in this approach. An evaluation of the centre produced in 2005 by the University of Central Lancashire is more wide-ranging than CAHHM's study and gets to the essence of Bromley by Bow's strengths and weaknesses.[9] It saw that the arts programme had worked across all the centre's activities to provide a dynamic, 'an ability to "pitch in" and get things done, and for a reflective and evaluating frame of mind'. This dynamic ensures that the centre combines what it terms 'inner world' work with external outreach and community development.

The Bromley by Bow Centre demonstrates the broad skills mix in community health delivery that was called for in the Wanless Report (2001),[10] and it could claim to have pioneered the Health Trainers initiative from the mid-1990s. By 2004, however, its groundbreaking approach to community development had foundered in some respects. The University of Central Lancashire researchers see this as a result of political tension arising between the aims of outreach work and the concept of the centre as the community itself and its 'communal ownership'. They also noted some inherent conflict between the medical training of GPs and the Bromley by Bow Centre's ethos – but the medical staff who have reconciled this tension see the advantages and support of multi-professional working that is relationship-based. The pace of development, however, has allowed too little opportunity to reflect on practice. The report's chapter on health concludes:

> A central premise is that encouraging people to meet and build relationships creates energy. This is backed up by art which calls inner resources into play and aids communication across difference. But our evaluation also shows the deep levels of cultural change which are needed to bring about such integrated working and the great amount of initiative, reflection, mutual support and resourcing involved in sustaining it.[11]

It is possible that the Bromley by Bow Centre has been over-ambitious. Without its charismatic leader Rev. Mawson (now Lord Mawson), who moved on in 2000 to set up the UK's Community Action Network, the organisation has struggled to sustain its holistic focus just as its activities have mushroomed. Its many practical achievements, however, still make Bromley by Bow Centre a powerful exemplar of how the arts can work in a complex community development arena.

The tensions that arose from Bromley by Bow Centre's exponential development were also evident, though to a lesser degree, in the other four projects in the CAHHM study. Inclusiveness and sustainability in arts in community health go deeper than issues of demography and funding partnerships; rather they are key to a sense of ownership, mission and vision that provide the very springboard for the arts engagement. Researcher Angela Everitt concludes with the observation that:

> Perhaps one of the most significant findings of this study is the newly emergent professional practice around arts in health in community settings. Community artists are occupying a very important space concerned with immediate responsiveness to 'problems of living'; the development of innovative, participatory solutions within relationships of equality and respect; and the prevention of more intractable situations. It is vitally important that this space is resourced and is protected.[12]

Attention to the quality of relationships forged through the work is paramount, because that inherently is both its strength and fragility.

## ISSUES AND THEMES FOR ARTS IN COMMUNITY HEALTH

Characteristics of practice emerge from issues that help or hinder the work, and they also reflect themes that arts in health is drawn to address. Exploratory audits that I did of arts in health activity in North East England and Yorkshire[13] and in the East Midlands[14] reviewed the work of around 50 arts in health organisations, and, based on information gleaned in semi-structured interviews, they revealed common perceptions and concerns.

There is an eagerness to share reflection on practice, so it is frustrating that there has been little opportunity to do this at conferences on arts in health, as they tend to focus primarily on hospital-based practice and take the form of retrospective case presentations rather than collaborative inquiry. The thematic strands that emerged from speaker presentations at the Dublin International Conference on Arts in Health in 2004, for example, were ones that arts in community health could readily engage with, even though they were primarily articulated in the context of arts in healthcare environments. I would like to run through those themes and suggest how arts in community health could have been affirmed in the conceptual base of that conference's agenda – because I think the Dublin event was a landmark in what conferencing in this field should aim to represent and achieve. More illustration of these themes will be provided later in the chapters of case examples. The identified conference themes at Dublin, produced in a report by CREATE,[15] are described here.

➤ *The notion of home* – This is also a central concept in arts in community health, shaping meaning and identity for participants from collective creativity, locally perceived health needs, the creation of congenial workspace, celebration, extended family and a domesticity of approach and atmosphere. As the biologist René Dubos observed, home is not so much a physical place as a psychological space with which our deepest emotions are connected.[16] In healthcare environments, 'the notion of home' is more specific to design; Bryan Lawson and Michael Phiri's evaluation study[17] of new hospital buildings, for example, noted the importance for patients' recovery of having a domestic atmosphere in their surroundings.

➤ *Healing and curing* – This is more problematic for arts in community health, as it usually works on a wider agenda addressing the social determinants of health rather than with the individualised therapeutic processes more commonly found in arts in hospitals and other institutional healthcare settings. Claims to heal through the arts also set up very tough evaluation questions seeking clinical evidence to support the impacts claimed. Community arts can, however, build social integration, heal the divisions in communities that impact on health, motivate healthier lifestyle choices, alleviate stress caused by environmental factors and provide support in personal or collective trauma, e.g. bereavement.

➤ *Understandings of illness and health* – The Dublin conference focused particularly here on how arts can foster emotional intelligence and how attention to feelings-based quality of life may challenge the norms of how health and illness are defined. (It is somewhat surprising then that the conference report's discourse is concerned less with a social model of health than with a biomedical one.) In arts in community health, there is an increasing convergence of three sectors – arts, health *and* education. As the Wanless Report to the UK Treasury on future health needs observed,[18] literacy is the key determinant of health. Literacy could be extended to include emotional literacy, because when the practice of arts in community health works to a social inclusion agenda, a respect for difference and diversity and the nurturing of emotional empathy becomes a guiding ethos for the work.

➤ *The interrelationship between different forms of intelligence* – This conference theme presumably derives from Howard Gardner's theory of multiple intelligences, which argues that there are many more human capacities than those that conventional education systems develop.[19] Arts in community health projects can focus as much on the skills acquisition of participants as on indicators of health gain. A community arts technique such as lantern-making, for example, can draw a wide range of intelligences to bear, as evidenced by the frequent use of the activity in schools as a basis for cross-curricular studies. In community contexts, the most successful projects are those that lay down educational and social pathways to channel awakened enthusiasms.

➤ *The benefits to the artist and the art form* – Arts in health has opened new areas for social engagement by artists and has created interest in the inherent therapeutic qualities of arts practice, whether applied directly one to one in art therapies or indirectly through collective creativity around a health theme. Arts in health may also consider the effect of art on what psychologist David Smail, in *The Origins of Unhappiness*, has termed the 'pathology of the environment'.[20] As with any pioneering arts intervention, there is a need for artists to centre their thinking on what makes for good practice. The experiential learning of artists who are developing community-based projects that address health issues can help with devising appropriate training and induction methods for new artists entering the arts in community health field.

➤ *The necessity of art* – The conference speakers emphasised the necessity of art as a means of acquiring knowledge, initiating action, expressing meaning and maintaining balance and good health in both individuals and society, and as a means of causing healthy 'dis-ease' in challenging accepted norms about health. But the way that the conference considered all of this as an expression of health was a bit too inward-looking. It is equally important to address the community contexts in which arts in health occurs and in which people are tackling other necessities related to socioeconomic conditions.

At the Dublin conference, common themes subsequently identified in the 'How To . . .' workshops were able to focus down more on practicalities. These covered the themes that follow.

➤ *Elements of good practice* – The elements identified in workshop discussions comprised securing sufficient time and space, respecting individualisation, subverting power relations, creating linkages with the wider community, quality, duty of care, and evaluation. All of these are central to arts in community health. However, they are not separate elements; they are bound together to the process through which the work unfolds.

➤ *The effectiveness of the arts in addressing distress and dislocation* – The arts are seen as a positive distraction for those in ill health. This underscores the importance of providing congenial spaces for arts interventions, with an atmosphere of positive regard that addresses persons, not patients. It is not just about providing arts activity or distraction or about putting over health information creatively; it is also a process of transition that respects the dignity of persons, building trust and reciprocity within communities in an environment in which people are not just made to *feel* valued but are *truly* valued. It requires a high degree of engagement and openness to learning on the part of professionals working in collaboration with each other and with community members on a personal level. What goes on around the arts intervention is as important as the artwork itself.

➤ *The need for greater integration of arts and health* – I think the conference report is right in recognising here the need for a fundamental change in how we think and work in health contexts, and that this is what can fuel meaningful partnerships. It requires seeing the 'arts in health practitioner' as not just the artist but as a nexus of connected professional interests developing a shared agenda and practice. If, as the report suggests, arts in health is currently undervalued by both of these sectors and seen as a marginal activity, a way forward would be to test public support for it through those healthcare channels that are particularly aimed at achieving public participation – preventive health, public health and patient forums. Arts in community health can create constituencies of interest in this work.

The Dublin conference report called for a coordinating body to disseminate information, promote work in both sectors and lead strategic policy at national level. This seems a tall order for any one organisation, especially in an area of work that is still on a journey of exploration. An independent organisation similar to the UK's National Network for Arts in Health could advance the first two aims, but strategic policy would be out of its hands. A networking approach, however, may alleviate some of the difficulties arising from the lack of a national strategic approach to arts in health – a problem felt as much in the UK and Australia as it is in Ireland. I want to illustrate next an interdisciplinary approach to effective networking and partnership. This can also open up training opportunities for both arts workers and health workers that are directly linked into practice.

## AN INTEGRATED APPROACH – COMMON KNOWLEDGE

The need for effective, practice-based networking came to light for me in developing a programme called Common Knowledge, which was set up in 2000 as the arts in health component of the Tyne and Wear Health Action Zone. This initiative enabled CAHHM at Durham University to coordinate a major programme of experimental work using arts-based approaches to examine health over a four-year period. Common Knowledge aimed to draw together different perspectives in order to increase capacity for arts-based approaches to health by engaging artists, health professionals of all kinds, teachers, local government and the voluntary sector to devise and deliver imaginative health interventions.

   Health action zones (HAZs) were a time-limited government initiative that aimed to encourage a multi-agency approach to addressing health inequalities in areas of high socioeconomic deprivation. The Tyne and Wear region of North East England has traditionally had some of the worst health statistics in the country, aggravated by declining industry, health-impairing lifestyles and high unemployment.[21] Economically weakened urban areas like Tyne and Wear have been resistant to traditional approaches to health gain, requiring health services to accept a shift to understanding of the social determinants of health so that non-clinical perspectives are taken more seriously. The Wanless Report cited 1970s research showing that health services account for quite a small impact on overall health status, at most about a sixth.[22] Determinants with stronger health impacts include literacy, sanitation and income. (The strongest of these is the female literacy rate.)

An arts initiative was welcomed into the Tyne and Wear Health Action Zone programme by the chief executives of the two district health authorities, who were able to persuade their peers that the programme would benefit from a creative approach to addressing its key priorities of mental health, cancer, heart disease, older people and children, as well as contributing to an underlying aim to develop capacity.

Over four years, Common Knowledge evolved as a flexible, multilayered network of organisations and individuals connected by interest in the relationship between arts and health. It developed groups focused on localities, groups focused around specific art form applications (such as therapeutic uses of music) and care groups (such as the elderly with dementia). It could be seen as a tapestry of relationships woven together from different strands of discussion. Many individuals in the network also represented organisations. The network had a strategic layer that worked through a governance group, which included representatives from local authorities, the arts, education and health, and a constituency layer of representatives (i.e. people who had participated in events).

Common Knowledge was organically developed through the alliance of its members, requiring only two part-time coordinators to facilitate meetings and help set up 50 pilot projects in a wide range of settings. Artist and CAHHM associate Mary Robson, who led the development of this approach, describes Common Knowledge as 'not one grand construction but many small ground works'. There was continual reflection on the quality of relationships formed between participants in the programme in order to point up that it is not what we do in arts in health but how we do it that counts. The arts in health practitioner was seen as a collective rather than an individual. That perspective encouraged collaborative working between people from different backgrounds and relieved the burden on the artists to deliver the whole project.

Common Knowledge worked in real local contexts across the five local authority areas of the Tyne and Wear region to address such major questions as: What does health mean? How can engagement with the arts improve health status and lead to health gain? These were the guiding questions in a series of two-day induction events for up to 60 people at a time, which explored how different art forms might be applied to a range of healthcare and community health contexts. This induction was followed up periodically with day-long events termed 'six-hour coffee breaks', in which facilitated discussion groups, their composition determined by local geography or common interest in a health issue, developed ideas for pilot projects. 'Revelation days' were also held to explore new ways of working (examples included arts-on-prescription schemes, participatory evaluation and emotional literacy for health).

The network grew in its first year of operation to over 250 members. Time was built into the programme for reflective practice in order to share learning, evolve common purpose and minimise the kind of complications that Bromley by Bow Centre encountered.

In 2002 Common Knowledge ran a prototype arts in health campaign in health buildings and public transport systems across the region to celebrate the work, gauge public awareness of arts in health and delineate a structure that could make for genuine joined-up practice in future in this field. Artist-designed bill-board posters, their contents distilled from discussions by Common Knowledge participants, appeared in Metro stations across the region. Operating Theatre, a now well-established theatre group of GPs, medical students and actors, gave its debut performances at Live Theatre in Newcastle. On 1 May 2002 a region-wide event entitled 'One Day . . .' deployed street theatre acts and musicians in the main Metro and bus stations, ferry services and local hospitals. The enter-tainment was an 'icebreaker' for the handing out of artist-designed postcards depicting Common Knowledge projects with health messages. The key lessons from the day were that the medium can indeed be the message and that arts in health is a concept that the public can readily grasp.

Most of the 50 pilot projects developed through Common Knowledge were closely documented by their participants in open journals, and many of these present stand-alone insights into working on health issues via the arts. There are a wealth of stories that can be mined from them to help with understanding more about the relationship between art and health. Admittedly, the anecdotal nature of this evidence was an inherent weakness. The focus of research was not on the individual projects so much as on the collective pooling of insight, learn-ing and experience developed through the network. As Common Knowledge was able to evolve organically, the research agenda that underpinned the work was not predetermined; rather it became identified in the process of building those cross-sector partnerships that initiated the pilot projects. Figure 1 sum-marises how the programme was organised and how it evolved.

Because there are different concepts about and approaches to the practice of arts in health (sometimes even within the same project), it was important to establish where each pilot project sat within the diverse and complex field of arts in health in order to better understand what it was trying to achieve. Individual projects were evaluated with regard to their contribution to the development of the learning exchange network that increasingly characterised Common Knowledge's role as a resource for arts in health practice across the Tyne and Wear boroughs. The focus was less on the health outcomes of individual projects (time and budget prevented robust assessment of these) and more on

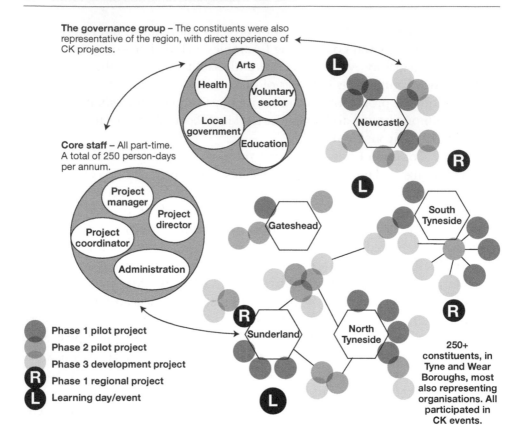

**FIGURE 1** The Common Knowledge network

the process of capacity-building for undertaking effective arts interventions in health contexts.

Evaluation of the Common Knowledge programme was carried out by Tom Smith of the Judge Institute in Cambridge. His observations of the induction events and local project planning led him to set out in his interim report (2001) a concept of the arts in health field as a diamond-like arrangement.[23] For participants, this proved a useful and accessible way of looking at the arts in health field, assisting the setting of aims and objectives for projects. The conceptualisation is not intended to be a definitive view, but rather suggested a way of exploring the multifaceted nature of health. Fundamentally, the diamond reflects the different ways in which health can be understood and the different ways in which a health intervention is viewed (*see* Figure 2).

In some ways the four corners of the diamond reflect the tensions within the field. In the top half of the diamond, creativity is the focal point of arts in health – but not exclusively. The arts can lead into discussion about communal and

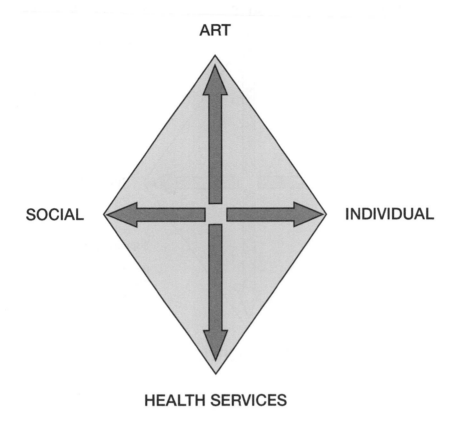

**FIGURE 2** Key dimensions of arts/health I

individual understandings of health. The arts on the top right of the diamond are understood as a health intervention in their own right. In the bottom half of the diamond, the focus of the arts in health activity is on the delivery of health services. The higher up the diamond, the broader the understanding and the more that creativity is seen as a health intervention. The left–right axis reflects a different unit of analysis, whether health – either clinically or artistically understood – is seen as an individual or collective thing. On the left-hand side of the diamond, arts in health activity is more focused on social relationships, within the community or between health services and people. On the right-hand side, the focus is more on the individual. Overall, the diamond reflects a philosophical orientation of the relationship of an understanding of health and the interventions to impact on health (*see* Figure 3).

Examples of Common Knowledge projects included: a Newcastle GP holding singing sessions for referrals to use voice as an alternative means of expression to combat stress (top-right segment); a project using writing and painting with

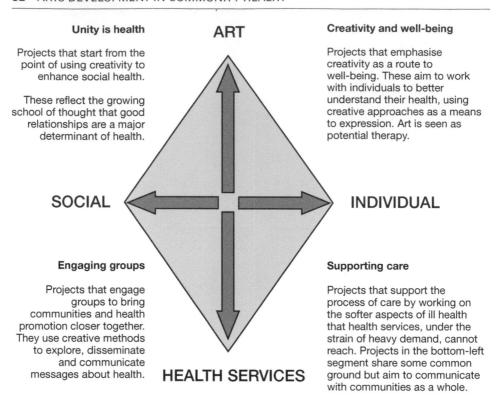

**Unity is health**

Projects that start from the point of using creativity to enhance social health.

These reflect the growing school of thought that good relationships are a major determinant of health.

**Creativity and well-being**

Projects that emphasise creativity as a route to well-being. These aim to work with individuals to better understand their health, using creative approaches as a means to expression. Art is seen as potential therapy.

**ART**

**SOCIAL**

**INDIVIDUAL**

**Engaging groups**

Projects that engage groups to bring communities and health promotion closer together. They use creative methods to explore, disseminate and communicate messages about health.

**Supporting care**

Projects that support the process of care by working on the softer aspects of ill health that health services, under the strain of heavy demand, cannot reach. Projects in the bottom-left segment share some common ground but aim to communicate with communities as a whole.

**HEALTH SERVICES**

**FIGURE 3** Key dimensions of arts/health II

cancer patients (bottom right); and a project working with the elderly with poetry and photography in order to understand their experience in care homes and stimulate collaborative activity between elderly people around a creative task – such as embroidery, painting or writing. These creative tasks can generate healthy discussion and engagement (top left).

At a national conference for HAZs organised by CAHHM in 2001, the (then) secretary of state for health, MP Alan Milburn, endorsed Common Knowledge, and he expressed an interest in approaches that would fall into the bottom-left quadrant of the diamond. In part this reflects health sector self-criticism – there is room for improvement in the way the health agenda engages with communities. The majority of Common Knowledge projects could actually be classified within this quadrant. Articulating the insights of this approach was felt to be important in order to develop thinking around a whole programme rather than just individual projects, and to enable those in the North East region, the rest of the UK and elsewhere with similar aspirations (and ideas which are not mainstream) to feel less isolated.

## MUSIC FOR HEALTH

This is an example of a Common Knowledge pilot project that addressed the right-hand side of the diamond, working in a health service context but also providing insights about the engagement of artists with people that could usefully inform community-based interventions. The ability of some projects to move across different sectors of the diamond is testament to their adaptability and strength, but it is important that the project knows at any one time where its activity sits within the field in order for appropriate research methodologies to be applied.

Music for Health came about as a result of a Common Knowledge induction event, where a cellist met a cabaret singer and got chatting with a GP who was keen to try out 'live' arts in her surgery. The GP was also willing to broker introductions to other healthcare settings for the musicians. Common Knowledge was able to provide some 'seed' funding to initiate a programme, and CAHHM wished to observe its potential for longer-term research. The musician who led the project, Tabitha Tuckett, has described it as follows:

> *Music for Health* began as a pilot project in community healthcare settings in Gateshead. We had two advisers: a GP and a nurse practitioner, and two musicians: a cabaret singer and myself, a classical cellist. As the project developed we performed music in waiting rooms, hospital wards, a care home and a general practice surgery, and covered many areas of healthcare including elderly care, mental health, stroke recovery, and learning difficulties.
>
> We performed only to those who said they would like some music, and our repertoire covered jazz, classical and folk music, show songs, local popular tunes and hymns. Not only patients but also visitors and staff asked for requests, often sang with us, and even taught us their favourite pieces. After this first project, we undertook a second in the intensive care unit at the Queen Elizabeth Hospital in Gateshead, in response to comments from staff that the unit often missed out on arts activities because of the perceived extra sensitivity of their environment.
>
> As a classical musician I was initially doubtful whether my music would appeal to many patients, but I soon learnt that patients' musical tastes are as various as their personalities. The number of people asking for classical pieces, whether or not they knew the title or composer, taught me that criticism of 'imposing' classical music on a social mix of people is itself patronising. All people have the ability and desire to enjoy all sorts of music including classical, as I learnt when someone with profound learning disabilities to our surprise showed little interest in the singer but asked for solo Bach on the 'cello to be repeated, clapping to the rhythms faster and faster and getting up to dance. She had no awareness that this famous music was often considered difficult or inaccessible.

Another aspect of the work that took me by surprise was how nerve-racking it is to perform to so intimate an audience. Unlike in a classical concert, your audience in a hospital bed will give you immediate and clear feedback about what they do and don't like, and each patient will have different tastes. We realised early on, from listeners' reactions to the music, that listening to live music involves participation just as crucially as making music, which would very often have been inappropriate. One elderly person had failed to talk or engage with people all morning, but after a song sat up alert and recalled memories of attending a dance nearby when young. On another occasion, the family of someone who was dying specifically asked if we could play and sing some favourite music for them just outside their room, and I hope that hearing our music made a very difficult time more bearable. A happier occasion was when we were able to perform some special requests for a husband visiting his wife in a long-stay setting on the day of their wedding anniversary.

This project has left me not only with a renewed impression of the emotive and communicative power of performing music, but also with a sense of gratitude to the patients, visitors and staff who gave us the privilege of making music for them.[24]

I later accompanied the two musicians – cellist Tabitha Tuckett and singer Margaret Frayne – into the intensive care unit (ICU). For several months the musicians had been providing a discreet music service on request for this ICU's staff, patients and their relatives. The initiative was now jointly supported by the hospital and Common Knowledge.

Some hospital staff had initially been understandably nervous about such a bold intervention, worrying that it might distract or disrupt care, or that it might even require communal participation (which for some seems a fate worse than death). Additional assurances were given to the hospital's ethics committee that there would be no breach of confidentiality, particularly in the journals the musicians were keeping to reflect upon their project as part of the evaluation being conducted through CAHHM.

Tabitha rang me an hour before the ICU session to confirm it would take place. Due to the sensitive nature of the location and the circumstances of the moment, less than half the sessions could take place as planned and the cancelled ones would then have to be rescheduled. It was felt that in future this pilot project, rather than being session-based, should look to become a residency, with the ICU having first call on the musicians.

My journal entry for this visit records the following:

Tabitha and Margaret meet me at 5pm and take me through to ICU. They are proudly bemused by their identity badges that proclaim 'NHS Musician'. We are greeted by the unit's nurse manager. She by now seems quite relaxed in having the musicians' regular 'recovery service' brought into the unit. She tells me how one of the nurses has been really excited by this project and is writing about the therapeutic uses of music as part of his degree course in critical care nursing.

This is the time of changing work shifts in ICU. Today is less busy than usual. Present are seven nurses, four doctors, a domestic, and four patients only one of whom is conscious. Tabitha unpacks her cello and uses an orthopaedic stool as a makeshift music stand. I shrink into a chair, suddenly nervous. Margaret stands in the middle of the floor. 'Start me off' she says, 'what should I sing?' I suggest 'something by Ol' Blue Eyes, but mellow'. And she's away singing a cappella *It's One for My Baby, and One More for the Road*.

Then Tabitha plays two Bach airs, Margaret joining her scat-style on the second one popularly known as the Hamlet cigar tune. (Somewhat ironic, I realise later, given the North East has the highest cancer rates in England. This hospital is also in a district with just about the worst coronary rate in the country.) They sing and play at a level just above room noise. And in the pauses between tunes, the chamber music of intensive care asserts itself like subdued Stockhausen – a constant hiss of gas cylinders, the occasional monitor bleep, and the clinical babble of staff quietly conferring. Everything here is as it should be – intense.

But the mood becomes more relaxed. The conscious female patient blinks recognition at the end of each number. Staff are preparing to move her to the High Dependency Unit next door. Tabitha tells me that at their last session all six beds were occupied. One old guy clapped feebly at the end of each piece, later confessing 'You don't know the good that's done me. See, I'm a musician too' – a heartfelt response as this is not a place for sentiment. At their very first session the musicians were asked by a family to play last requests for a dying relative.

Margaret encourages the staff to make their own requests. So we get *La Vie en Rose* and a medley from *Sound of Music*. Two relatives come in to attend an unconscious elderly man in a corner bed, while Tabitha is playing an Irish melody. The nurse manager enquires if they'd like the music to stop as they're clearly upset. No, they say, but ask if it could it be more upbeat. Tabitha obliges. The musicians are constantly judging the appropriateness of what they are doing, responsive to the medical teamwork and trauma going on around them. Every bit of this 'performance' is in a very real sense on the edge.

Visiting hours begin. A last song from Margaret, 'Shall I do *Every Time We Say Goodbye*?' Her mouth opens, then she checks herself, abashed. 'No, definitely not . . . try *Wonderful World*', and she's off again.

Afterwards during tea break in the staff room, Margaret says last week a young male patient asked her to 'do some Queen'. 'The only one I could think of was *We Will Rock You*.' 'Better than *Another One Bites the Dust*', quips a male nurse evincing the kind of humour you need to retain the sanity required of the

job. And I imagine that, her singing *'you got blood on yer face, yer big disgrace . . .
we will, we will rock you'*, transforming a macho anthem into a lullaby.

How do you put a value on work like this, identify its cost benefits? Some
ICU staff have anecdotally noted a reduction in blood pressure in coma
patients that has coincided with these music sessions. This could be the basis
of a longer-term research programme if it can raise resources and get Ethics
Committee approval. The essence of the intervention is already here in that it is
about sensitising and alleviating the clinical environment through the potential
pleasures of music in itself for people in distress, some in crisis. It is probably
the most extreme circumstances you could place the arts in, short of a war zone.
I am awed by the pluck and sensitivity of the musicians in taking on work as
challenging as this.[25]

In 2001–02 the Chelsea and Westminster Hospital undertook an in-depth
evaluation of the benefits of arts in healthcare,[26] focusing on the 'flagship' arts
programme developed there by Susan Loppert. Although this hospital has
always been regarded as the benchmark of quality in commissioning artworks
for healthcare settings, the study's early findings revealed that music had a higher
satisfaction rating than visual art among hospital staff, patients and visitors.[27]
The study team, led by Dr Rosalia Staricoff, went on to frame and explore more
difficult questions around clinical outcomes, with intermediate indicators
emerging to show that music reduced anxiety.

An evidence base for the effectiveness of arts in health could have a nar-
rowing effect, simply using rather than developing the art form in its context,
unless we can also achieve a better understanding of what makes for quality in
arts interventions in the clinical environment. Tabitha Tuckett's project revealed
that both the musicians and the music have their own unique subtlety if the
engagement is approached in the right way. She and Margaret Frayne went on
to deliver this initiative in two other North East hospitals and to train other
musicians to work in an ICU environment.

Tuckett's project began as a number of tentative 'taster sessions' in a range
of healthcare environments, some of them community-based, with mixed
success – a cello proved incredibly loud in a GP's waiting room, for example
– but later on moved into the most clinical of environments short of an
operating theatre, where it became increasingly valued by ICU staff as a welcome
diversion and boost to morale. They did not have a fixed repertoire to perform
but rather attempted to respond to music requests. On a later visit I made with
the musicians, a nurse was about to turn the musicians away when the ward
sister came up and said, 'No, we're having a hard time in here today. We need
you.' The musicians aimed to establish quickly a sensitive relationship with
patients, visitors and staff based on what they had learned earlier from offering
a personalised service in community-based contexts. This shows that there can

be some fluidity in a project to cross over different facets of the arts in health diamond, connecting practice and research across different tiers of healthcare.

## IT'S ON THE TABLE

This was a region-wide project that addressed the left-hand side of the diamond, developing creative health information and building community links. It's On the Table originated in discussions at local meetings that revealed there was a common interest in developing a project on the theme of nutrition. Someone brought a newspaper report in to the first meeting that described how a recent social trends survey (this was in 2002) indicated that two out of three British households no longer used a dining table. This became a prompt for discussion at the other local meetings and shifted interest away from nutrition to issues around social eating.

Uniform interest in this theme across the five boroughs of Tyne and Wear enabled Common Knowledge to undertake for the first time an art project that would collectively represent the network. In each of the five boroughs, three community groups were invited to work with a local artist in designing from coloured card a template for a decorative tabletop, working within common design parameters devised by artist Bridget Jones. These were then passed on to a furniture maker, who translated the design into wood marquetry using a corresponding palette of dyed wood veneers. Each table was of the same dimensions, with folding trestle legs enabling the tabletop design to be displayed on a wall at each group's home venue, rather like a shield or painting. Each table had an inlay section to accommodate an additional two-dimensional artwork, made by the artist alone or with the group, covered with Perspex to maintain the integrity of the table surface. The participating groups ranged from nursery-school children through to pensioners' groups, and the inlaid artworks encompassed embroidery, weaving, painting, photography, ceramics and metal engraving. The table designs were grouped under five themes – 'seeds, roots, shoots, leaves and fruits' – each one depicting the makers' view of the values and foods that made for healthy social eating.

The tables, which could accommodate up to six people, had a slight curvature so that they could be linked together to form a composite round table or helix. This was how all 15 tables were displayed in an exhibition at the Customs House in South Shields in 2003. Smaller groups of tables were later shown at health conferences throughout the North East. The tables stimulated discussion between the different community groups in Tyne and Wear who had made them, enabling them to have lunch together on occasion and share opinions and ideas for collaboration in arts in community health. The artwork thus became a concrete symbol of the Common Knowledge approach.

The interlinking of an artwork or theme across different participating groups helped shape the partnership ethos and delivery of projects within and between the five boroughs. Figure 1 (above) illustrates how in the final year or phase three of the programme, projects were pooling resources to develop a joint idea. An example of this is elderly care homes in three boroughs that employed the same group of artists to develop music and recitation events in their day rooms, with training for staff to continue the work. Another example is projects in South Tyneside that decided to develop the social eating theme further in schools and primary care contexts. One GP clinic in that borough, for example, worked with a digital artist to design a laminated card providing a hieroglyphic summary of key reminders for self-care management of newly diagnosed diabetes patients. This was later republished for national distribution.

## LESSONS LEARNED FROM COMMON KNOWLEDGE

Although HAZ funding for Common Knowledge expired after three years, the programme continued for a further year with charitable trust support to attempt to embed the approach and the shared learning. The overall network slowly dissolved when its part-time administration stood down in 2004, but threads of connection formed from some participants' personal journeys through the programme persist to this day and have influenced further project development. Common Knowledge has influenced, for example, the health strand of the Creative Partnerships programme of North and South Tyneside, which will be considered in the case examples in Chapter 7. It could be useful in the evaluation of this type of programme to track the participants both within and beyond the network in order to determine what connections it helped establish and what learning had been absorbed and applied elsewhere. A longitudinal study would therefore attempt to measure change not only in participants in arts activities but also in those developing and delivering the activities.

From 2005 CAHHM went on to adapt the Common Knowledge approach in the development of a learning network for arts in health in the East Midlands, but here it focused more on providing learning days and mentoring of individual projects. The network developed out of an audit of practice in the region in 2004 and out of the formulation of an action plan commissioned by ACE and the Directorate of Public Health East Midlands.[28] This arts in health network is integrated into a larger regional public health network known as Emphasis.[29]

Difficult lessons were learned in the early years of Common Knowledge about the governance of this kind of network and its relationship-based approach. Tensions arose, sometimes to the point of culture clash, between the core team, who provided the part-time administration with a focus on facilitating the development of a guiding ethos for the programme, and a steering group that had been set up at the outset of the programme and whose membership was selected on the basis of geographical and sector representation. The main problem was that most members of this steering group, who held managerial posts in their own sectors, did not actively engage with the programme but considered that their role was to monitor it on behalf of the HAZ.

The situation was eased in 2001 when it was agreed that the core team would be based in CAHHM at the University of Durham, and that CAHHM would also administer the grant support (it had previously been administered through one local authority on behalf of all five). This gave Common Knowledge more independence and greater accountability. The steering group then agreed to stand down in favour of a governance group drawn from a cross-section of participants in the actual programme. Decision-making on the direction and content of the Common Knowledge programme was henceforth made by this new group. This relieved the pressure on the core team that arose from a feeling that they were being held to account by a select committee rather than having a support group with firsthand knowledge of the programme.

At its outset Common Knowledge set ambitious aims to:
➤ mutually define arts in health for the Tyne and Wear Health Action Zone
➤ create a positive emotional environment for the programme
➤ change the way that people work.

Tom Smith's interim evaluation notes that Common Knowledge made progress in advancing the first two aims, but that against the third aim, 'the majority of its impact is at the micro rather than macro level; for example, Common Knowledge is influencing the way people work locally but finding it more difficult to do this at a strategic level.'[30] He later perceives that this problem originates in an ideological tension that comes to the fore in evaluation:

> The differences between arts and health should not be overplayed, but under-stood. There will always be tensions between the two fields. Perhaps the most important is epistemological. The two regard empirical data and its analysis in quite different ways. For this reason the credence given to aspects of experience (in arts-led practice and evaluation) makes forming a common pool of knowl-edge a difficult challenge.[31]

Although it is possible to achieve a cross-sector consensus on the purpose and process of delivering arts in community health, it is difficult for that pool of on-the-ground experience to flow uphill into executive decision-making. Differing views may emerge on what constitutes an evidence base for target-driven strategic thinking. This will be explored further in Chapter 8, on evaluation.

A sense of working against the grain is a commonly felt frustration when evaluation is applied as a challenge rather than a stimulus to arts in community health. The Australia Council for the Arts' report *Art and Wellbeing* draws similar conclusions to those of Smith on Common Knowledge:

In considering the role of community cultural development, it is useful to distinguish between *instrumental* approaches which involve the arts ('let's implement policy using the arts') and *transformational* approaches ('let's allow creative activity to determine policy, negotiate shared understandings and map out solutions').[32]

I suspect a combination of both approaches is required, though there would be an inclination in arts in health practitioners for a weighting towards the latter, with its focus on empowerment. When an instrumental approach is prescribed by health services, arts are regarded more as a minor tool to achieving health aims rather than as a transformational catalyst.

It appears that a programme such as Common Knowledge can thrive in a climate of permission where health services engage in exploratory partnerships to tackle health inequalities, but the lack of abiding sanction means it can only formally last as long as the temporary initiative, and it thereafter depends on the covert conversion of participants to another way of working. At this point the open exchange of viewpoints developed from a forum approach is compromised, and reflective practice becomes restricted to personal professional development rather than being a reflexive means of achieving and evaluating collective working. To re-form a network, you must wait for a chance to get arts through the back door of the next government health initiative. A means to circumvent this déjà vu may lie in the drawing up of a code of practice, though this has so far proved to be problematic also.

## TOWARDS A CODE OF PRACTICE

With an aim to harmonise working practices of artists and health professionals, some early attempts have been made to establish a code of practice. For example, the Greater Manchester Arts and Health Network *Code of Practice*[33] (2005), which borrows heavily from a general code of practice devised earlier for visual artists,[34] states that good practice in arts in health consists of the artist's knowledge, skills and attitudes to:

➤ *Contribute Confidently* by engaging with the development of ideas, and solution of problems, by refusing to pigeonhole and to be pigeonholed, by challenging stereotypes and assumptions about who knows what, by being generous with their knowledge and their skills, by knowing their worth.

➤ *Prepare Thoroughly* by finding out where, with whom and how they will be working, by researching context, legislative implications, location, environmental concerns, potential impact, and interests of partners and colleagues.

➤ *Collaborate Creatively* by establishing mutual respect and recognition, through identifying shared goals, encouraging the views of others,

welcoming open and informed discussion, valuing complementary skills, co-operating and collaborating in achieving a vision without losing sight of their own identity and integrity.
➤ *Aim High* by aspiring to bring quality work to everything they do, whether presenting ideas, managing professional relationships, negotiating or producing the work.

In conjunction with this, health and well-being good practice is seen to consist of the readiness to:
➤ *Adopt Professional Accountability* by understanding the need to respect the rights, dignity and autonomy of every person through maintaining confidentiality and obtaining informed consent, knowing the limits of their practice and when to seek advice, demonstrating effective and appropriate communication skills and behaving with integrity and honesty at all times.
➤ *Adopt Planning and Strategy* by using research, reasoning and problem solving skills to determine appropriate actions, knowing the importance of evaluating research and evidence to keep informed and be able to audit, reflect on and review practice.
➤ *Adopt an Informed Approach* by being aware of common health and well-being methods, artistic applications and new developments through regular networking and understanding of other Arts and Health professionals' work, building and sustaining multidisciplinary relationships and being able to establish and maintain a safe and effective practice environment.

I think the problem with a code of practice like this one is that it is mostly directed at the artist, supplementing the requirements for a competent arts practitioner with a whole raft of extra responsibilities relating to governance, research skills and partnership management that have to be 'adopted'. I think rather that these are responsibilities that should be shared by project partners, with a support structure in place that enables the artists to concentrate on engagement with participants and delivery of the project, while allowing their input on the health and well-being aspects of the project to be contributed and valued. If this code of practice were translated into a job description, it would probably run to several pages. It shows the range of skills ideally required to undertake arts in community health, and there is inevitably a shortage of artists with this breadth of knowledge and experience.

The acid test for a code of practice is whether it can actually translate into practice in the field. This particular code was proposed at a time when LIME, a key arts and health delivery agency for Greater Manchester, was attempting to roll out a citywide programme called Pathways with a complex web of partners;

and the wider North West region, through Arts for Health at Manchester Metropolitan University, was preparing to deliver an ambitious Treasury-funded Invest to Save programme that would develop capacity in the workforce and link projects in a common evaluation framework. In LIME's case, on-the-ground experience showed that too much was already being required of artists too soon, and adopting a code of practice on these terms would have only formalised the problem further in a one-sided way.

LIME's Pathways programme was a three-year arts initiative developing referral processes to promote mental health and well-being in the community. It was an exploration of creative solutions to mitigate the social exclusion caused by mental ill health, and it involved artists working with local people to find ways of overcoming emotional difficulties and daily stresses. The stated aim was to uncover meanings for terms like 'well-being' and 'quality of life' among the target groups. Integrated referral pathways were researched and explored in the first phase of the project, and two specialist artists, a drama worker and photographer, were commissioned to explore creative ways of engaging people and working with the issues raised in the second phase. The first phase of the project started in August 2003 in Wythenshawe, a housing estate with high levels of social deprivation. The second phase, with the aim to roll the programme out across the city, started in May 2004. The project was a partnership between LIME, Manchester City Council and the South Manchester Healthy Living Network.

Although the project achieved its numerical targets and produced artworks of a high standard with participants, the delivery of the programme was dogged with problems. An interim evaluation gives a refreshingly honest account of what went wrong.[35] This is a thorough, probing and honest report that identifies problems that are common to arts in community health, and its attempts to address these without hyping up the qualitative evidence of success is admirable.

Pathways was funded principally through a Neighbourhood Renewal initiative which, with its complex partnerships and delivery targets, may not have been conducive to an exploratory programme like this. The lack of an on-the-ground coordinator to support the artists was a problem, but the difficulties may have been in the partnership framework itself. The problems the report identified go to the heart of current practice and research. They are as follows:

➤ establishing effective referral mechanisms with local health services
➤ the tension between individual therapeutic and social outcomes and the proper role of the artist in helping produce these
➤ the development of arts-led evaluation, and who interprets this and how
➤ achieving participatory evaluation.

The project attempted to use some creative techniques to assess participant response, using picture icons rather than scales to indicate the participants' moods, but these had mixed results and could not be collated statistically. If an evaluator had been present when these arts-based evaluation tools were administered, it would have flagged at an early stage the paucity of usable data. Perhaps there should have been more process documentation, but the fragility of the groups and the necessity for the artists to multitask inhibited this.

Prominence was given to asking participants experiential questions, such as 'What have you found out about yourselves?' This could have set Pathways in a learning-development context, but this would require a more supportive relationship to be built up between artists and participants than the session-based activity would allow. It is the sort of questioning that is difficult to just drop into a session-based format. Perhaps the emphasis should have been more on collective creativity and end products than on individual exploration of feeling.

The referral mechanism is outlined in the report more as a set of principles than as a practical route, and it seems too loose. In practice it needed to be more disciplined, with a step-guide for referrers, and it failed to ask what the criteria were for assessing suitability for referral. The project showed that groups very quickly became 'closed', with no capacity to take new members. So the nature of the projects themselves needed rethinking, as they did not square with the referral principles.

An insightful comment in the report is that 'we felt that what we perceived as an inward looking, therapy-oriented approach might militate against the potential of artistic processes that can create something that can be shared with others.'[36] This is central to the arts therapy versus arts in health debate and prompts consideration of what kind of art intervention is appropriate and what is the ethos of sharing. This project, like many others, struggled to articulate what 'well-being' means in arts in health.

As Pathways entered its second phase in 2004, it needed to assess how it was weighted in terms of the instrumental or transformational approach. It was apparent that the Neighbourhood Renewal framework was still locking the project into the instrumental approach, making it difficult for the artists' perspectives to be embedded in the research and for the arts activity to be regarded as more than a 'tool'. A second Pathways report, produced by the Research Institute for Health and Social Change at Manchester Metropolitan University, suggests that fault lines in the programme's first phase, e.g. artist counselling and supervision, were being addressed by the end of the research period.[37] Processes of referral to the arts activities were still problematic, however, with resistance in some of the established arts groups to taking in new members. This reveals the downside of the 'bonding' rather than 'bridging' form of social capital.

An artist's observation in this report that 'the whole is more than the sum of its parts' is crucial – it needed time and mechanism for all agencies involved to reflect on process, share learning and own a bigger programme than their individual project goals. In the latter phase, workforce development proved as important as delivery, building the inclusion aim on the experience of the partners themselves. As with Common Knowledge, the ethos was seen to begin with 'us', not 'them'. An effective code of practice might thus evolve from joint aspiration based on agreed values rather than just instruction to the perceived delivery agent.

If there is a common weakness in the arts in community health programmes I have described in this chapter, I suspect it lies in the tension between frontline engagement and back-room strategic direction. When projects are successfully networked together, there is a momentum of learning development and organic growth that can challenge the initial assumptions on which the programme partnership was formed. In this field of work, no one can stay on the touchline. It invites immersion in the process, but it also requires continuous review. Before formulating a code of practice, it might be better to establish and agree the underpinning principles of the work.

## SEVEN ESSENTIAL PRINCIPLES FOR ARTS IN COMMUNITY HEALTH

I use 'for' rather than 'of' in this section heading because I hold that there are certain principles of creative activity that may result in what can be described as arts in community health, but they are not *a priori* attributes of a particular arts technique. Effective practice is significantly reliant on sensitivity to context and the quality of the interaction with participants.

The first principle I see in this work is recognising art as a gift rather than a commodity; recognising that it is something created for an occasion to exchange information, feelings or experiential wisdom. I referred in the last chapter to Lewis Hyde's *The Gift*, an anthropology-based account of how art is shared in the public realm. Hyde sees in particular how art is most potent in collective creativity that builds integration through the act of giving. He says that:

> Reciprocity, the standard social science term for returning a gift, has this sense of going to and fro between people. When the gift moves in a circle its motion is beyond the control of the personal ego, and so each bearer must be a part of the group and each donation is an act of social faith.[38]

The use of circles earlier to diagrammatically describe the processes of Common Knowledge and the Bromley by Bow Centre is more than metaphorical; it illustrates the nature of arts development as a gift exchange in the promotion of community health. Reflective practice is also frequently depicted as a cyclical process.

The gift is also a recognition of the innate talents of the participants and that everyone has something to contribute. Health comes from individuals realising their potential and gaining access to other opportunities for personal and social advancement. This is what I term 'the social tonic'. It is character-building for the individual, and it can also increase morale in the social group: the 'look what we did' factor. When cultural activities in arts, sports and community action can clearly show that the people involved in them are valued, they stimulate a reciprocity that other kinds of public-sector intervention struggle to achieve, and so they are central to a regeneration strategy, not just window dressing.

The second principle is the creation of congenial space. This is not just a physical space but also a climate for meaningful engagement where conversation comes naturally. Instrumentalised approaches to arts in health tend to underestimate the importance of this, looking for effects without care for the process. The therapeutic qualities in making art are enhanced by the social interaction and conversation they stimulate, and the transformation of a space to a place of temporary celebration is the very manifestation of collective creativity. Congenial space is defined by John Angus as:

> a spirit of high energy, laughter, purposeful and excited creative activity and the beginnings of trust, credibility and confidence. This space is a privileged ground between a community's potential for action and change and its alienated and deprived members. It is an embryonic focus for well-being. It is also, hopefully, a space where health and social workers can meet community members on their own terms.[39]

The third principle is responsiveness in being able to identify and address health needs at the same time, valuing the participants' contribution in producing art relevant to their situation but also challenging them to assist in creating work that provides a quality experience. Responsiveness thrives in a climate of continuous positive regard. To be more than simply a 'smiley' culture, however, responsiveness also needs to be informed by reflective practice as a foundation of purposeful learning – taking a perspective on one's own actions and examining experience rather than just living it.

A fourth principle is fostering self-care as a learning process. A model for this may be found in 'complexity theory', which is gaining increasing interest in the field of management of chronic illness. Helen Cooper and Robert Geyer, for example, apply the theory to self-care management of diabetes, where the acceptance of complexity can provide a structure that allows for both traditional and complementary therapies.[40] They show that the development or 'emergence' of adaptive behaviour is characterised by:

➤ self-organisation
➤ the ability to be able to deal with new problems as they arise
➤ the ability to connect things together to make sense of what is, accepting that life can at times seem chaotic
➤ recognition of the fact that perfection is not always possible, so mistakes will happen.

I can see that these rules apply equally to how we learn and make art. Cooper has commissioned artwork in the past that helps explain the onset of diabetes to newly diagnosed patients, and she now sees that:

> Art has a place in the traditionally scientific evidence-based world of medicine, particularly when the success of treatment depends upon patients' self-management practices and not just expert advice . . . [it] provides a place where one can 'see' how all the bits and their interconnections fit together.[41]

A fifth principle is affirming identity and a sense of place for individuals and for communities. Both sickness and intervention can produce dislocation, and what community-based arts in health can provide is a reintegration of self through supportive communal creativity. Making art together can be a relational practice that helps participants to achieve or regain a sense of their social abilities. This has implications for social inclusion in areas of high health inequalities that are characterised by a paucity of social capital, low expectations and disenfranchisement through apathy. In addressing these problems, issues of identity and place become paramount, and the picture is more subtle and complex than epidemiology statistics alone can convey. It may be useful to explore whether in different socio-geographic situations there is a common experience of what makes an 'unhealthy' community and how local arts development can improve health literacy.

A sixth principle is to generate well-being from an enhanced sense of community. This may take different forms. A report from the Globalism Institute in Melbourne[42] classifies three kinds of community: 'grounded community', found in tangible face-to-face settings; 'way of life community', which builds social capital from common attitudes and lifestyle; and 'projected community', which creates temporary or virtual environments in which to model new possibilities. Well-being, it states, has become more than physical and mental health, in that 'our social and communal world is not simply the contextual background to our wellbeing but rather fundamentally constitutive of it.'[43] As well-being is increasingly seen to be a prime determinant of social value, it poses a political challenge far greater than the already difficult problem of sustaining equitable health and medical services.

The seventh principle is fostering a sense of responsibility. Michael Wilson's factors that make for health, which form the epigraph of this book, constitute the spectrum of well-being in the public realm, and at the high end is responsibility.[44] A publication from Disability in the Arts, Disadvantage in the Arts Australia (DADAA) presents an interesting perspective on this in an artist's reflection on the benefits of her using a community mental health arts studio:

> One of the things about mental illness is that you don't take responsibility until you manage your illness. This place gives you a lot of opportunity to show responsibility. Because you will let people down if you don't hang an exhibition. You would let friendships down. This place is like another home. You have an opportunity to take responsibility and it is really good for your health.[45]

Here a therapeutic benefit is sensed from a combination of autonomy and obligation to others, and this revelation derives also from a sense of having found 'another home'.

When these generic principles are translated into characteristics of practice, they may appear to be unique to each project, because they reflect personal journeys of engagement and creative effort. 'Making special', to use Ellen Dissanayake's term for vernacular art-making, is dependent on particular occasion, place and congregation.[46] I shall be returning to consideration of principles, themes and characteristics of practice in the next four chapters, which present a number of in-depth case examples. These are mostly drawn from participant observation, and to some extent they recount a personal journey in the making of this book.

## REFERENCES

1 Lindstrom B, Eriksson M. Contextualising salutogenesis and Antonovsky in public health development. *Health Promot Int.* 2006; 21(3): 238–44.
2 Antonovsky A. *Health, Stress and Coping.* San Francisco: Jossey-Bass; 1979.
3 Health Development Agency. *Art for Health: a review of practice in arts-based projects that impact on health and well-being.* London: Health Development Agency; 2000.
4 Arts Council England. *The Arts, Health and Wellbeing.* London: Arts Council England; 2007. p. 20.
5 Hacking S, Secker J, Kent L, *et al.* Mental health and arts participation: the state of the art in England. *J R Soc Promot Health.* 2006; 126(3): 121–7.
6 Health Development Agency, op. cit.
7 Everitt A, Hamilton R, White M, editors. *Arts, Health and Community: a study of five arts in community health projects.* Durham: University of Durham (CAHHM); 2003.
8 Ibid. p. 17.
9 Froggett L, Chamberlayne P, Wengraf T, *et al. Bromley by Bow Research and Evaluation Project: integrated practice – focus on older people.* Preston: University of Central Lancashire; 2005.
10 UK Treasury. *Securing Our Future Health: taking a long-term view* [the Wanless Report]. London: HM Treasury; 2001.
11 Froggett, Chamberlayne, Wengraf, *et al.*, op.cit. p. 85.
12 Everitt, Hamilton, White, op. cit. p. 77.
13 White M. *Determined to Dialogue: a survey of arts in health in the Northern and Yorkshire regions.* Durham: University of Durham (CAHHM); 2002.

14 White M. *Seeing the Wood for the Trees: an arts in health action plan for the East Midlands.* Durham: University of Durham (CAHHM); 2004.

15 CREATE. *Report on the Dublin International Arts and Health Conference.* Dublin: Arts Council Ireland; 2004.

16 Dubos R. *So Human an Animal.* London: Hart Davis; 1970.

17 Lawson BA, Phiri M. *The Architectural Environment and its Effects on Patient Health Outcomes.* Leeds: NHS Estates; 2003.

18 UK Treasury, op. cit.

19 Gardner H. *Multiple Intelligences: the theory in practice.* New York: Harper Collins; 1993.

20 Smail D. *The Origins of Unhappiness: a new understanding of personal distress.* London: Constable; 1993.

21 North East Assembly. *State of the Region.* Newcastle: One North East; 2001.

22 McKeown T. *The Role of Medicine.* London: Nuffield Trust; 1976.

23 Smith T. *Common Knowledge Interim Evaluation Report.* Durham: University of Durham (CAHHM); 2001.

24 Tuckett T. Personal communication.

25 White M. The power of music. In: Bolton G, editor. *Dying, Bereavement and the Healing Arts.* London: Jessica Kingsley Publishers; 2008. pp. 124–5. Reprinted by permission.

26 Staricoff R, Loppert S. Integrating the arts into healthcare: can we affect clinical outcomes? In: Kirklin D, Richardson R, editors. *The Healing Environment: without and within.* London: Royal College of Physicians; 2003. pp. 63–80.

27 Staricoff R, Duncan J, Loppert S, *et al.* A study of the effects of visual and performing arts in healthcare. *Hosp Dev.* 2001; **32**: 25–8.

28 White, *Seeing the Wood for the Trees,* op. cit.

29 www.emphasisnetwork.org.uk (accessed 18 August 2008).

30 Smith, op. cit. p. 6.

31 Smith, op. cit. p. 83.

32 Mills D, Brown P. *Art and Wellbeing.* Sydney: Australia Council for the Arts; 2004. p. 9.

33 Greater Manchester Arts and Health Network. *GM Arts & Health Network Code of Practice.* October 2005. Available at: www.wlct.org/gmahn/cop.pdf (accessed 4 August 2008).

34 Corner L. *Code of Practice for the Visual Arts.* Artists Information Company. 2003. Available at: www.a-n.co.uk/knowledge_bank/article/92660 (accessed 5 January 2009).

35 Storey R, Brown L. *Pathways: an evaluation of the pilot phase.* Manchester: LIME; 2004.

36 Storey, Brown, op. cit. p. 58.

37 Sixsmith J, Kagan C. *Pathways 06: project evaluation final report.* Manchester: Manchester Metropolitan University; 2006.

38 Hyde L. *The Gift: how the creative spirit transforms the world.* New York: Routledge; 1979. Republished Edinburgh: Canongate; 2006. p. 16.

39 Angus J. *An Enquiry Concerning Possible Methods for Evaluating Arts for Health Projects.* Bath: Community Health UK; 1999. Republished Durham: University of Durham (CAHHM); 2002. p. 25.

40 Cooper H, Geyer R. *Riding the Diabetes Rollercoaster: a new approach for health professionals, patients and carers.* Oxford: Radcliffe Publishing; 2007.

41 Ibid. p. 76.

42 Mulligan M, Humphery K, James P, *et al. Creating Community: celebrations, arts and wellbeing within and across local communities.* Melbourne: Globalism Institute RMIT; 2006.

43 Ibid. p. 25.

44 Wilson M. *Health is for People.* London: Darton, Longman and Todd; 1975. pp. 59–60.

45 Lewis A, Doyle D, editors. *Proving the Practice: evidencing the effects of community arts programs on mental health.* Fremantle: DADAA; 2008.

46 Dissanayake E. *What is Art For?* Washington: University of Washington Press; 1988.

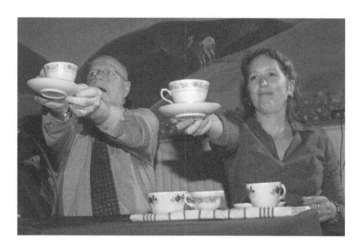

MOMENT, Cork Capital of Culture 2005. PHOTO: CORK FESTIVAL OFFICE

# CHAPTER 4

# A change of seats: case examples from Cork, Ireland

Changing of seats from far to near.
A melody, a harmony,
Humming then awing,
Soon there is music in every ear
But that is not all that is happening here.

Excerpt from a poem by a participant in the Music in
Healthcare/Mental Health project – part of the Cork Capital of
Culture 2005 *culture + health* strand.

In Chapter 1 I described how I first became involved in community-based arts in health when I was working for the celebratory arts company Welfare State International (WSI). That first project took place in a small GP practice in the West Midlands in January 1988. At the same time, the company was working on a much bigger initiative in Glasgow, which culminated in an event on St Mungo's Day, 13 January, at the city's cathedral. Here, in the worshipful company of assorted clerics, planning officials, news crews and the Lord Provost in full regalia, WSI helped choreograph a procession of inner-city schoolchildren accompanied by the police pipe band over the Bridge of Sighs by the Necropolis to the great door of the cathedral. It was an extraordinary pageant, fusing elements of Pied Piper mediaevalism, Blake's *Holy Thursday* and state-of-the-art PR. St Mungo, Glasgow's patron saint and first bishop, was to be 'guest of honour' in a peculiar iconography.[1]

WSI artists had been invited by the City Chambers to assist with the order of the day. The company's main contribution was to create and present two complementary gifts to the dean at the inaugural ceremony for a sheltered housing development in the cathedral precinct. The first gift was a handcrafted 'seed' lantern (depicting, in a totemistic way, the life of St Mungo), intended to lay the ground for a three-year WSI project to turn Glasgow into the 'City of Light' when it celebrated its distinction of becoming European Capital of Culture in 1990. The second gift was a steel canister in the form of a spire, encasing a hermetically sealed time capsule to be buried under the cathedral forecourt. Inside this capsule were children's stories, drawings and architectural fantasies for the future of their city.

Back in the cold January of 1988, a tentative artists' residency in a Midlands GP surgery and the civic pomp of that Glasgow parade seemed to be totally unrelated projects, connected only for me as the launch events of WSI's twentieth anniversary year. Yet over time the two projects have merged in my mind as a pointer to the direction of arts in community health.

Each year a city or sub-region in one European Union member state holds the prestigious title of Capital of Culture. This designation is awarded to countries in turn, and they are then given the opportunity to invite their cities to compete to host the festival. In 1990 Glasgow used its Capital of Culture status to revitalise both the infrastructure and character of the city and developed a successful model for a socially-focused festival programme rather than just a high-art jamboree. Much of the outreach programming was channelled through the Glasgow City Council's Social Work Department to deliver a key festival aim of achieving social inclusion on a massive scale within a cultural context. That department's annual budget for arts activities rose from £25 000 to over £1 million in two years.[2]

Fifteen years later, when Cork in southern Ireland held the Capital of Culture title in 2005, it took Glasgow's example for inspiration but focused on a partnership with health services rather than social work. Cork was a pathfinder for the orientation of arts in health to address itself not just to individual health contexts and communities but also to cities and their citizens. When Liverpool took up the mantle of Capital of Culture for the UK in 2008, it too made culture and well-being a major theme of its programme.

### *CULTURE + HEALTH* FOR CORK

As part of Cork's festival preparations, the Capital of Culture organisers developed a wide-ranging programme titled *culture + health* to connect healthcare settings, arts centres and the community at large. The main festival programme aimed to extend its reach of exhibitions, performances and artist residencies into healthcare settings, as well as coordinating specific health-themed projects with target groups such as the elderly and clients using mental health services. In conjunction with the region's Health Service Executive (HSE), the festival office established a fixed-term arts in health post to deliver the programme.

I made two brief visits to Cork in Autumn 2005 to try to absorb the impact of the *culture + health* strand within the varied facets of Cork's health and social care infrastructure. In just those few days, I was able to sample the dress rehearsal for a multimedia performance work in a sheltered housing unit, a puppet show by residents of a long-stay hospital and local students, an international poetry reading on hospital radio, a specially commissioned play in an elderly persons' care home, a display of fabric art by children with dyspraxia, tree dressing in the grounds of a hospital chapel and a folk concert in a mental health unit. I also took in some mainstream festival events that had lateral connections to the exploration of health themes, such as the 'Home' exhibition at the Crawford Gallery. And outside the Opera House, I witnessed the cathartic extreme sport of 50 teenagers who were head-banging their way through Beethoven's *Ode To Joy*.

Between these events, I gave talks on the practice and research of arts in health to mixed audiences of arts, health and social care professionals. This did feel, however, like bringing coals to Newcastle, or rather from Newcastle, which is close to where I live. Because culture and health had been such an integral part of the Cork 2005 European Capital of Culture programme, the city was already as ahead of the game on arts in health practice as anywhere else I could think of.

My title for this case example derives from a poem by a participant (who later trained to become a music facilitator) in the Music in Healthcare/Mental Health project at St Stephen's Hospital in Glanmire. The line 'Changing of seats from far to near' seems to sum up both the context and achievement of the *culture + health* strand in the Cork 2005 programme. It speaks of inclusion, confluence, empowerment and an engagement with the arts that is personalised through the creation of a congenial space for its enjoyment. But as the author writes, 'That is not all that is happening here' – the outcomes have been as wide-ranging as the programme itself.

The *culture + health* strand was an ambitious initiative comprising three key projects, 10 artist residencies and over 20 smaller, yet no less significant, performances, workshops and events. The residencies also provided training in different art forms for care workers and other HSE staff. For example, two seven-week blocks of training linked to residency activity revealed latent talents in care staff, especially musical, and this enables some of them to continue to deliver activity to their clients beyond the 2005 programme. The Cork 2005 Office had set up a working group with the health and social care sector to oversee the programme and determine its legacy through a sustainable and holistic approach to arts in health.

Despite the exponential growth internationally in arts in health practice in recent years, Cork did something that nowhere else had so far attempted; it articulated the relationship between arts and health services throughout a city and its environs, and it built the potential and vitality of such a relationship on the involvement of those who might otherwise be marginalised due to their health status. The brightest legacy that a Capital of Culture designation can offer is a renewed confidence and cohesion, notable not just in centres of cultural excellence but also in centres of necessity – in hospitals, care homes and social services settings, both formal and informal. The Cork 2005 Office also did a relatively simple thing that built on the example of Glasgow in 1990 – it consistently facilitated access to its mainstream events programme for people dependent on care. Other festivals could learn from this.

*Culture + health* recognised a developing orientation of community arts, cultural education and outreach services to the addressing of health issues. The international conference on arts and health held in Dublin by Arts Council Ireland in June 2004 took stock of what was happening in Ireland and elsewhere and set out an agenda for its future development.[3] In alliance with the HSE Southern Area, Cork 2005 aimed to advance that agenda and show the relevance of local arts development to current health policy. Up until then, arts in community health programmes in Ireland had been confined discreetly to a few local-government-supported arts initiatives, such as an intergenerational arts in health programme in Sligo begun in 2000[4] and a nationwide network of small pilot projects developed by community arts agency Blue Drum in 2004. Both Music Network Ireland and the Waterford Healing Arts Trust were also developing models of participatory arts in institutional settings that could have application in wider community contexts.

As Orla Moloney comments in an evaluation of a Music Network Ireland programme:

> Organisers and practitioners worked in isolation and there was no sense of belonging to a coherent 'arts and health sector', let alone an opportunity to collaborate in the development of a national arts and health policy. The activity that has been taking place in the arts and health sector across Ireland over the last five years has begun to highlight the value of the work for all stakeholders involved, and to address some of the most problematic issues facing it. Diverse projects were devised at local, regional and national level in order to break the isolation of those involved, and to develop models that would contribute to good practice in the field. At city and county level, for example, a number of local authority arts offices and regional arts centres devised and evaluated innovative programmes facilitating artists to gain valuable experience and develop specialised skills in the field. At national level, the Arts Council published an Arts and Health Handbook (2003) and hosted an international conference on Arts and Health (2004).[5]

The Cork 2005 festival was arguably the first arts initiative of national profile to address a health policy agenda. Its *culture + health* strand provided a clear example of how the arts can engage in the partnership approach advocated in the Irish government's *Quality and Fairness* health strategy.[6] That report's foreword, written by the (then) health minister, Micheál Martin, MP for Cork South, stressed the importance of addressing health inequalities caused by poverty and disadvantage and noted that 'the strategy at all points envisages cross-disciplinary collaboration to achieve new standards, protocols and methods.'[7] The report recognised that many other factors, and therefore many other individuals, groups, institutions and public and private sector bodies, have a part to play in the effort to improve health status and achieve the health potential of the nation. The strategy acknowledged that cultural conditions can impact on the social determinants of health and required the formal and informal roles of family and community in improving and sustaining well-being in society. It concluded that the quality-of-life aspect of health needed to be highlighted, and that this would involve creating a supportive environment to maximise social well-being for vulnerable groups.

Using the arts to help develop that supportive environment in the context of a city and region is a considerable challenge, and it required a diversity of work in both healthcare and social settings. Some of the *culture + health* projects in 2005 focused on the intrinsic therapeutic benefits of the arts, others focused on environmental improvements to support health staff in delivering their care services, and still others looked at producing more creative approaches to achieving patient-centred care. In addition, there was community-based arts in health work tackling issues of social exclusion and focusing on a concept of social capital. The programme thus addressed the four principle areas of arts in health as described in the Common Knowledge 'diamond' diagram in Chapter 3.

For Cork 2005's *culture + health* project manager, Ann O'Connor, 'the year was one of nurtured and informed experimentation', but only in the aftermath perhaps was it possible to reflect on what had really been achieved. There was recognition that the programme had been a learning process for all involved.[8] As a member of the Cork 2005/HSE Working Group for the strand commented to me, 'The strength of this programme is that there has been a huge respect for the competencies and skills and peculiarities of all our fields.' Such a sharing of perspectives infused the coordination as well as the actual delivery of the projects. It established a confident base for cross-disciplinary research, coupled with patient involvement, that I believe should be the way forward in the evaluation of arts in health.

Firstly and rightly, the *culture + health* strand placed patients and HSE clients at the centre of the work, and through their participation in creative activities it sought to celebrate their relationships with staff, carers and the wider public. This was a bold move, for often with arts in health the safer recourse is simply to commission artworks and performances for healthcare settings. A combination of both approaches seemed to signal that a momentum was being generated in all involved to continue this work well beyond 2005.

## THE *CULTURE* + *HEALTH* PROGRAMME: SOME PROJECTS AND OUTCOMES

The appropriately titled Encounters project was a unique partnership developed between two organisations from the arts and health sectors – Triskel Arts Centre and St Finbarr's Hospital. This partnership gave the artist coordinator, Charlotte Donovan, the opportunity to evolve a calendar of quality artist residencies, workshops, installations and events throughout 2005. Early in the year, she took the time to develop relationships with staff and patients as a precursor to any art activity so that attention could be given not just to the artwork itself but also to how it enhanced the daily life of the hospital. 'I didn't approach this as *my* residency,' she told me, 'but as something *we* want to happen'.

An arts-led open day on the feast of St Finbarr in September gave thousands the opportunity to experience the hospital as a living community, rather than as an array of clinical and rehabilitative units. It also overturned the hospital's design limitations in identifying indoor and outdoor spaces that could provide a patient-centred environment for both personal and communal contemplation and enjoyment. It relieved the sadness that many felt about the place, partly due perhaps to its workhouse origins, and instead affirmed the best qualities of an old-style, community-based hospital. It was not only the image of the hospital that was improved. As the head of nursing observed, 'This artwork is health promoting, and it's keeping the patients alive. It is providing a vitality that is as crucial to health as treatment.' The hospital secured funds to continue the programme in 2006 and to extend the project's activities out of the hospital into the city, thus making it the hub of community outreach work.

Sustainability of course cannot be built on enthusiasm alone; it also requires reflective assessment of the impact of arts interventions in health and indicators of their benefits. Music Network Ireland's evaluation of its project in Cork was crucial to its aim to establish a model of good practice for music in mental healthcare settings. This project was based in St Stephen's Hospital, Glenmire, and the Carrig Mór Centre, Shanakiel. The combination of direct observation, reflective practice by the musicians and testimony gathered from staff and patients at St Stephen's and Carrig Mór suggested that key benefits of the participatory music sessions were a fostering of empathy and self-esteem among participants and the restoration of 'a sense of individuality that is often lost or damaged when a person suffers from mental illness'.[9] The methods of engagement and evaluation in Music Network Ireland's programme were adapted from a model that it had developed in its earlier partnership with the Midland Health Board (MHB). That model facilitated group tuition and live performance in residential and day-care environments for older people (nearly 300 participated) within a context that addressed the MHB's mission to maintain the independ- ence of older people by improving community services. After an initial pilot phase, the MHB committed itself in 2002 to supporting a three-year action research project, in which a mentoring scheme for the musicians was set up from 2003. Music Network Ireland was able for most of the project's duration to employ a full-time education and healthcare manager to work closely with a counterpart in the MHB, although funding difficulties later on resulted in less successful staffing arrangements. Funding also restricted the activity to six-week blocks in each care setting, highlighting a need to find ways of not dissipating its effect in the intervals between sessions. Orla Moloney was able to apply the learning from this project to her evaluation of music development work in Cork in mental health settings.

The Midland project had encouraged older people to engage actively and creatively with skilled musicians. Ongoing evaluation noted and tracked outcomes such as improved relaxation and concentration in older people with dementia or memory loss, improved motivation and mobility, and feelings of self-esteem and community integration amongst the participants. Mentoring assisted the musicians to appreciate the role and benefits of music in the wider community. In some cases the project changed the way that care staff regarded and worked for their clients, though in other cases it highlighted confusion over roles and responsibility of care staff during the music sessions. Quality was considered crucial to the success of the activity and became closely linked to a sense of dignity in participation. From early on, however, attempts to undertake quantitative evaluation were frustrated. The collection of feedback gleaned from the forms given to participants at each session was inconsistent, so data could not be collated quantitatively. Furthermore, other evaluation measures introduced independently by the MHB frustrated a joint assessment of data. The partnership proved strong in opening access to funding streams within the Department of Health and Children, however, and the view from on the ground was that the pooling of different professional expertise to deliver the project was greater than the sum of its parts. It demonstrated how the cross-sector working that is encouraged in the Irish government's Health Strategy could be effectively achieved, and it addressed elements of the *Adding Years to Life and Life to Years* report[10] that call for facilitation of creative opportunities.

Moloney's report lamented that there are 'very few opportunities to network with others involved in similar structures in order to optimise the learning and avoid the pitfalls already identified', and she concluded:

> No national policy for arts and health exists and in its absence initiatives such as the *Music in Healthcare* partnership are exposed to changing priorities and interests in both the arts and health sectors. While the *Music in Healthcare*

project feeds into the national aims and objectives of each sector, it has not been prioritised in terms of funding and resources in either. There are a number of reasons for this. Firstly, the arts and health sector remains unorganised and largely invisible. Secondly, the nature of the work makes it difficult to document and promote and as a result, there is insufficient regard for its value at every level. Thirdly, because it straddles two sectors, policy makers from each can assume that the other should be responsible for its development. Arts and health is a small and vulnerable area of work. With no policy back-up, the two agencies have struggled to attain adequate resources.[11]

In order to sustain the achievements of the project, the report recommended that the partners consider moving the project on to a musician-in-residence model, also drawing on local music expertise and community links. It also called for them to collaborate on any future evaluation processes from the beginning. Orla Moloney told me a key problem she identified was that however strong the arts and health partnership is, when key personnel change or move away the project falters. This suggests that even strategically directed programmes remain heavily reliant on the personalities of their champions and the on-the-ground relationships they nurture. This is why networking is important in ensuring that knowledge of a project is widely shared, not vested in a few individuals.

This model that Music Network went on to refine in Cork allowed patients to access their own innate musical skills and exercise artistic choice within a context of collective creativity. To help identify such impacts from the perspective of both clients and staff, Music Network's researcher concluded that a participatory approach to evaluation, with clarity of aims and objectives, would be crucial. The challenge for future research into a project like this is whether that first step to choice can lead to greater autonomy and restored health of mind. For research to be meaningful, however, there must be continuity of the activity to assess its impact over time. The *culture + health* strand used its key projects as frames on which the health services could weave connections with other arts groups, both professional and amateur, with consideration from the outset of what would make for the sustainability of the initiative.

When I visited the Carrig Mór Centre at Christmas time, the Cork Singers Club's session in the day room was concluding with a rousing Pogues song, *Fairytale of New York*, with staff and patients in fine voice. Such celebrations were actually heir to a much older custom. In the late nineteenth century, Cork Asylum boasted a 20-strong band led by a professional bandmaster. A local newspaper report from 1876 on the band's Christmas concert noted that:

> The ballroom is a spacious and lofty apartment, and has recently been painted and decorated with artistic skill by the inmates. A splendid band is directed by an efficient bandmaster. Dancing, singing and other amusements are indulged

in, and this treatment has from long experience proved more effectual in
restoring the senses than the more stern procedure of close confinement.[12]

So arts in health is by no means a new venture for Cork. There are many similar
examples of health institutions in the UK and US that have a long history of
engagement with the arts. The difference nowadays is that whereas they once
simply made good sense, public spending pressures and accountability now
require that they prove their validity to the arts funding system and clinical
governance.

Another artist residency project was that of Molly Sturges, a director, com-
poser and performer from the US. Her work explores the intersections of music,
movement, performance and community-building. Under her direction, the
MOMENT project brought together a group of artists working in a variety of
media (dance, painting, writing, film, music and drama), who collaborated with
the staff and older people in the O'Connell Court residential centre and with
young people and adults from the local community. Commencing in June 2005,
the project challenged conventional barriers between art production, community-building and performance, what Sturges described as 'an engaged ensemble',
and culminated in a multi-site performance/installation in the autumn.

MOMENT was perhaps the best-realised example of a participatory arts
in health project asserting its quality and relevance to both contemporary art
practice and person-centred care. Over three months, the carefully nurtured
relationships between artists and participants developed organically into a
performance piece that was part-reminiscence and part 'live' art. As one staff
member observed, 'It came alive, grew out of abstract things . . . and created a
kind of family.' It drew the incidental details of participants' everyday lives and
recollections into a creative exchange with artists working in different media to
produce a shared experience that celebrated and astonished. The radiance of the
performers made it clear that the whole process had been great fun. MOMENT
had an artistic rigour that at first may have mystified the participants but in the
end proved revelatory. As one member commented, 'You want more of it – you
don't want it to stop.' It challenged and briefly changed ingrained patterns of
care management and mundanity, leading one care manager to declare that 'It
elevated minds to things other than survival here.' There were also identified
health benefits for some participants, such as less frequent visits to the doctor,
less medication required and more regular sleep patterns.

MOMENT can only live on through its dissemination and the individual
benefits it may have left residents and staff in O'Connell Court. Ideally, it could
have toured to other care homes in the district, building the confidence of its
ensemble cast to continue beyond a one-off project. In the process of making
MOMENT, it was difficult to predict its outcome; because community-based arts
in health projects often are characterised by 'informed experimentation', it is

common for them to only realise their potential and the research agenda that could inform them at the close of the work. This further argues a need for their sustainability so that they are not diversionary entertainments but pathways to improved health and social integration that can meet the needs and raised expectations of participants.

The energy and resources that went into Cork 2005's *culture + health* strand delivered a palette of possibilities that goes beyond the albeit vast confines of a year-long international festival. The deep immersion of arts into healthcare settings sparked a cross-sector dialogue for continuation of the work, so the finale conference in February 2006 was actually more like a prologue. In taking stock here of what had been achieved in the year, it seemed evident that the key projects, the artist residencies programme and the 20 or so smaller initiatives that took place had laid the groundwork for a vibrant network of arts in health activity around the city. The sheer diversity of practice and context in these projects brought arts in health practice into alignment with arts for older people, disability arts, arts for special-needs groups and arts in education. Having these connections at grassroots level should place the city's arts sector in a stronger position to address 'joined-up' policy-making initiatives at government level.

Several of the artist residencies had an integral training element, which sought to build connections between artists, health workers and community representatives, thereby redefining the 'arts in health practitioner' as not being just the artist but rather a network of people keen to explore a health issue creatively. A focus on resource development underpinned the delivery of the arts activity itself.

Dance facilitator Jo Nichols' A Time To Dance project, for example, took place in a number of settings where elderly people receive health or social service support. The project involved a team of dance tutors, who were in most cases also healthcare staff and community workers. As the project developed, the team evaluated and analysed its work. A notable observation was the surprise of many healthcare staff at the agility, enjoyment and concentration of older people once they got involved. At the end of the project, the lessons learned and the guidelines for good practice that were developed were fed back to a wider peer group of 27 dance tutors. The project alerted dance resources and care services in the region to what can be offered to elderly residents – and it achieved this on a modest budget.

Similarly, a project in the outlying district of Cobh, facilitated by Sirius Arts Centre, trained a women's group to facilitate visual arts work in a day-care centre. It established clear health aims within the district's regeneration agenda. The lead artist, Marie Brett, helped develop facilitators' skills in project management and reflective practice, providing them with a strong grounding in arts in community health. The artworks emerged naturally out of the learning relationship forged between the apprentice artists, day-centre staff and older people. The five collage canvases that were produced map the journey of the project and embody the revitalisation of the Cobh district through the eyes and handiwork of its senior residents.

Cobh Regeneration was an exemplary project and created a domestic familiarity around the art-making. My experience of arts in health projects elsewhere has taught me that this is the magic ingredient of good practice in this field. As a daughter of one of the Cobh participants told me, 'It has given my mam dignity. I can feel the heart in the works.' Dignity conferred through communal attainment in the arts has been a palpable social outcome of arts in community health. It also affirms why maintaining and enhancing a culture of person-centred care through the arts can be an important adjunct to health services.

Even an ephemeral experience of creative engagement, when it touches on the personal, can have a resounding impact. What most impressed a staff worker on the puppetry project in St Raphael's Centre in Youghal, for example, was 'the gentleness of it'. This project, the MOMENT production and others in the programme built intergenerational links between care institutions and local schools, providing a mutual learning experience that fostered a positive regard between the young and the vulnerable.

The *culture + health* strand prompted critical reflection by many health professionals who had been involved in it, because it brought into the open patients' and clients' views on services provided to them and the very meaning of health, and indeed the meaning of culture. The projects themselves also helped democratise this process, and the development of a forum theatre project with people with disabilities called Finding a Voice was an example of effective consultation on service delivery and improvement. This project, based in St Laurence Cheshire Home, enabled and facilitated the residents to articulate health and social care issues that mattered to them. Forum theatre could also be seen as a metaphor for the cross-sector collaboration that fuelled the *culture + health* strand. In forum theatre, you participate not only as an audience member but also as an actor or director, as you bring your unique level of expertise to bear on the issues identified by the group.

What I think worked best in the *culture + health* strand is that it did not require the arts to demonstrate their worth to healthcare at every turn; rather it examined the value of the relationships built up through arts activity between staff and the public. It signposted the benefits rather than the instruments, and so allowed the quality of the art produced to speak for itself.

## ART IN HEALTH IN CORK POST-2005

After holding a national conference to showcase the *culture + health* programme in early 2006, a new phase for the arts and health programme was established by HSE South. It aspired to build on learning from work undertaken in 2005 and from other initiatives taking place nationally and internationally and to advance this work in a strategic and innovative way. The creation by HSE South in 2006 of a position of arts and health coordinator indicated that there was confidence within the system to drive this work forward.

By 2007 the programme was working across all departments in the HSE to develop and deliver participatory arts activities, environmental enhancement, health promotion, research, training and networking initiatives. As part of this work, more participatory music workshops took place in regular eight-week blocks in the Carrig Mór Centre and St Stephen's Hospital. A similar music project was piloted at Cúnamh Day Hospital and at the GF Acute Unit at Cork University Hospital in 2007. Planning also began with South Lee Mental Health Services to develop a community-based music project in the Togher and Ballyphehane area.

The HSE South arts and health programme wanted to facilitate the sharing of ideas and learning from these projects within the workforce, so it applied for funding from the Health Services National Partnership Forum and was successful. The project aim was to build on analysis and learning from previous arts initiatives in mental health settings in order to deliver arts training and participatory arts workshops (with a focus on music) that could improve the quality of working life for multidisciplinary groups of staff and improve the quality of service delivery for service users in a variety of mental health settings. Objectives for the project were identified as follows:

1   to deliver arts training and participatory music workshops to staff and service users in five mental health settings
2   to focus on the experiences and needs of staff in each setting while also building on previous work with service users
3   to facilitate staff to meet and exchange ideas, solutions and challenges with their colleagues in the other four settings
4   to explore best models of staff learning and participation through workshops
5   to evaluate service user and staff satisfaction
6   to design a process for adaptation and transfer to other health settings.

I was then asked by HSE South to undertake a short evaluation study of the Cork Mental Health Arts Programme Music Initiative in spring 2008.[13] This was an opportunity to review the progress since 2005 of the mental health strand of the programme in respect to both workforce development and service delivery. The focus of the study was simply to assess how far the music initiative had been able to meet its aim and objectives.

There were significant external administrative constraints on the music initiative from the outset, and these are important for understanding the context in which the project operated. The grant was less than half of what had been asked for and was released three months later than the funder's timeframe originally indicated, leaving only two months to quickly deliver the project within the calendar year, as required. A more measured delivery period would have allowed for more reflective practice by participating staff, with better opportunity to explore the relevance of the project to issues of staff morale, retention and union relations. Although the intent was to keep the prime focus on the musical intervention's contribution to the quality of working life, a lot of management attention was absorbed simply in meeting the imposed tight deadlines for delivery of the session programme in each setting.

What helped to keep the project to its original aim was the effectiveness of the Partnership Working Group (PWG) regularly attended by staff from all five settings. A willingness in this group to listen, share in discussion and achieve consensus helped shape a common ethos. However, each mental healthcare setting was also encouraged to deliver and interpret the project as it felt appropriate, so each could have objectives additional to those of the overall project. Thus the GF Unit focused on patients who resisted participation normally, Cúnamh Day Hospital focused on self-expression and the Togher project concentrated on combating social isolation. Both Carrig Mór and St Stephen's Hospital saw the programme as an opportunity to consolidate work begun during the Capital of Culture festival in 2005 to achieve the inclusion of patients in arts opportunities that the city offers.

The programme uniquely covered the gamut of mental health settings, from secure wards to day care, thereby attempting to demonstrate its relevance across different tiers of service provision. Pivotal to the development of the programme were two learning days organised for a wider pool of staff and musicians. The second of these, which I attended, facilitated group reflection on the programme to date and then focused on a group exercise working through practical ideas for staff to facilitate their own sessions. The health professionals and musicians clearly held each other in positive regard; the word 'privilege' was repeatedly heard with reference to their joint participation in the programme. There was a sense of common ownership of the programme and a consensus on the wish for it to continue. As one community nurse manager commented, 'Ireland has tremendous ability in music, and this should flourish in the health system as it does in community.'

There were five professional musicians engaged on the programme, two of whom worked in three settings, one in two settings, and two in one setting. The musicians checked in with staff before and after workshops to jointly prepare for the session and debrief afterwards. The musicians met together twice during the programme to reflect on the impact of the work on their own practice; the main benefit cited by them was the experience of working in a team with other musicians and healthcare staff.

The musicians' 'exit strategy' has been to give staff a core activity they could lead for themselves, accommodating their different skills, capacities and interests. This aim arose because in the previous music initiatives the staff attempted to maintain the activity themselves between the eight-week blocks of session, with varying results. St Stephen's, however, proved an exemplary success, discovering it had good amateur musicians on staff, with one ex-inmate leading the facilitation of sessions after external training that included an MA in Community Music. Although sessions at Togher ran for only six weeks, this community-based project in a day centre produced a good band.

At Carrig Mór and St Stephen's, the participating staff members were able to judge what makes for appropriate and effective practice as their appreciation of music in a healthcare setting grew. That experience appears also to have peer influenced staff in the other, newer settings who were looking for creative solutions to their own needs. Staff on the GF Unit, for example, wanted to find alternative forms of engagement with patients that could make a difference. I heard staff from all five settings affirm that the music intervention had therapeutic benefit for themselves as well as patients, addressing both professional and personal needs.

At the PWG meeting I attended, someone made the passionate observation that 'A fire was lit in people. I could see arts and expression are vital to psychiatric care. Music gave hope to patients and staff.' I was intrigued by the reference to 'hope' and to arts intervention as a vital need, and I invited explanation. One member of the group said that 'Different therapies have different "languages". We must recognise that patients can be poor communicators. It is connection that gives hope. Music helps sense the mood in non-communicators.' Another helped to ground the discussion by declaring, 'Music is a basic communication tool. It doesn't need talent and formality. It is good for very ill people, because they can stay with it. It's a non-stressful discipline, but maybe it's impossible to evaluate? It's certainly a stepping stone to more complex interaction.' One person made the potent comment that 'It allowed a spirit and the unconscious to flourish.' This is not how one might ordinarily expect work in a mental health institution to be described, but it speaks volumes for the transformative knowledge that may come from a creative approach to training. It was clear that the music initiative had motivated staff to reflect upon and redefine the core values of the service. The environmental effect of the music was often instantaneous: 'It was a better place to be after the sessions.'

The PWG spoke of a need to have a different working atmosphere, one that is better suited to relationship-based working. Music seemed to help because 'It made the work environment different, it wasn't clinical or sterile.' But there was also concern that to outsiders and clinical superiors the intervention could appear superficial or contrary to governance: 'The clinicians' concern is "will anything go wrong here?" There are issues, for example, about documentation, but we don't have to be stiff about it. Most clinicians don't take it seriously.'

Prior to the PWG being established, its members had previously only met informally, if at all, and there was a perception that only the managers from different units would meet up to discuss operational matters and policy. The PWG conferred status on the project and provided a meaningful context for exchange of professional views and experiences. Members clearly took pleasure in how they had been able to enthuse each other to engage with the music programme, one describing the fun of it as 'incomparable'. It was gratifying to them that staff from other units had visited the project and taken part, and that the project would be promoted in forthcoming conferences at national level. Comments were made on how the project had developed confidence and job satisfaction, so participation in the music programme raised expectations in staff as well as in clients. An observation that 'It has provided self-efficacy and we have become champions of the work' was tempered with a reflection that 'Maybe now we have to leave behind those who don't want to change.' While this impacted positively on their perception of the work environment, it did also suggest an 'us and them' stand-off.

The programme coordinator told me at the time of application that she did not think managers would normally support an arts project, but they might be interested in this case to see how it would address staff issues. The issues subsequently identified (and addressed) in the programme included effective team working, better understanding of clients' needs, job status and satisfaction, training in how to lead participatory activities, workplace improvement and on-the-ground innovation versus senior staff scepticism.

The participating staff affirmed the value of being in a multidisciplinary learning programme. They felt the music initiative was ideas-rich, that it empowered staff to engage with patients less formally and that it provided an alternative to clinical intervention. Some felt that more clarity is needed in the model, however, in distinguishing between art and art therapy, as this can be confusing for both staff and patients. What appeared to attract patients to the activity was that it was not individual therapy but a pleasant communal diversion. Staff from Carrig Mór commented on the importance of the social inclusion element in the activity and referenced the benefits of the arts to mental health that are cited in the National Economic and Social Forum report on mental health and social inclusion.[14]

Project logbooks were kept at each setting. They functioned mainly as open comments books and did not differentiate between clients, staff and musicians. All the logbooks had useful observations, but one or two were especially well maintained and rich in data, including a record of attendances. Here are some of the comments:

➤ I was able to relax very well afterwards.
➤ The beat was great. It cheered me up and it is good for my depression.
➤ I look forward to coming and feel great afterwards.

➤ Room was too small for the crowd but can't wait till next week.
➤ It took my mind away from the problems I am dealing with currently.
➤ I spend so much time thinking, I find music is a great escape. You can almost see people losing themselves in the rhythm.
➤ Very uplifting and soothing.
➤ People felt free and encouraged to get up and dance.
➤ They really knew how to get the crowd going and give us a good time.
➤ It was good therapy on a Monday morning.
➤ I'm here early and looking forward to seeing everyone for the morning's session.
➤ I don't want to lose my place.
➤ The group was very well run and always had a friendly and welcoming atmosphere.
➤ Hope the music group will continue for a long time to come.
➤ I feel really honoured to have joined in the group here. I particularly felt the interaction of staff and clients and felt that I was part of something very worthwhile.
➤ I used to look forward to every Monday morning for the last six weeks.
➤ Music flowed throughout the corridors creating a distraction and a sense of serenity.

Satisfaction with the music activity stemmed from different sources – some saw its therapeutic benefit and others its impact on social connectivity, and many comments suggested the music was a special event in the healthcare settings' calendar, providing an experience within which people could bond. It could also help clients engage more proactively with their treatment plan; as one nurse observed, 'The activity helps patients to get into real therapies.'

The significance of patients' comments in the log book was particularly noted by staff at Carrig Mór: 'Even small comments are significant with this group. It opens conversation between staff and patients, gives triggers to discussion. It is possible to talk about other things than health problems. Otherwise the medical model prevails in all conversation. Instead we should be asking what is behind people's creativity. If the health aim is to heal the split in a person's psyche then connection with that person is vital.' The 'triggers to discussion' provided by participatory music-making were thus seen as an important step in each individual's road to recovery, enabling staff to get to know the person, not just the problem.

There were almost no negative observations of the programme by staff, only suggestions for improvement and concern that ending the project would confound patients' expectations. It was noted that new admissions at St Stephen's could be afraid of the group and needed more gentle induction. For some it could seem awkward and 'cheesy' when Irish standards and old-time ballads were played; but still, as one community nurse manager observed, 'It develops concentration and connection – it's the best thing I've ever seen for concentration.' One staff member of GF Unit came up with the most down-to-earth indicator of clients' engagement: 'They always come back into session after toilet breaks!'

The challenge to sustain the programme with less money after expiry of the grant raised concern for quality and professional approach, but some encouraging steps were taken by individual healthcare settings in the programme. The Family Centre agreed to work with the Togher Mental Health Association and run more sessions in their premises. It was felt that this would improve the partnership at local level, and other service budgets were identified by the partners to support continuation of the music sessions. The Family Centre put time and money into the initiative so clients' whole families could take part in future. The advantage of having the work occur in smaller neighbourhood settings meant that everyone knew about it. People often came into the clinic just to ask about future sessions. The GF Unit used Lotto money to support more sessions, and Carrig Mór offered placements to music therapy students, who would combine the music activity with training. It was felt much more could be done if senior staff would only approve and champion the initiative.

There are many similarities with the Common Knowledge approach in what has been achieved in the music initiative in Cork, including the gathering of basic data in project logbooks, which was a staple tool in Common Knowledge. The music initiative also forged a unique identity and purpose in bringing together the different tiers and institutions for mental health in the city and county. With a little more development it might have been possible to set out an integrated pathway for music-making in mental health services from institutional care to day services and into the community post-discharge. There was a risk, however, that the music-making might shrink back to becoming therapy rather than being community-focused. There was also less sense of the programme being connected with the whole city, unlike during the Capital of Culture festivities in 2005.

The programme had a specific focus on the impact of arts in health initiatives on staff relations within the work environment, but it is a pity the grant support was too short-lived to enable this to be explored more fully. The programme coordinator, Ann O'Connor, went on to a post as arts in health advisor at Arts Council Ireland, and her new role was to include drawing up a 'code of practice' for artists working in healthcare settings. This could help design not only the process for adaptation and transfer of projects like this into other settings but also the ethos by which they are done.

## REFERENCES

1 White M. Resources for a journey of hope: the work of Welfare State International. *New Theatre Q.* 1988; **15**: 195–208.

2 McCabe M, McVicar E. *Streets, Schemes and Stages.* Glasgow: Strathclyde Regional Council; 1991.

3 CREATE. *Report on the Dublin International Arts and Health Conference.* Dublin: Arts Council Ireland; 2004.

4 Moloney O. *HE+ART:* a participatory arts and health strategy for Sligo. Sligo: Sligo Arts Service; 2007.

5 Moloney O. *Evaluation of the Music in Healthcare Project 2000–2004: a partnership project between Music Network and the Midland Health Board.* Dublin: Music Network; 2005. p. 1.

6 Department of Health and Children. *Quality and Fairness: a health system for you.* Dublin: Department of Health and Children; 2002.

7 Ibid. p. 3.

8 Cork 2005 European Capital of Culture. *culture + health Strand: a study of 32 projects in diverse healthcare settings.* Cork: Cork 2005 Festival Office; 2006.

9 Moloney O. *An Evaluation of the Music in Healthcare/Mental Health project for Cork 2005.* Cork: Cork 2005 Festival Office; 2005. p. 15.

10 Department of Health. *Adding Years to Life and Life to Years: a health promotion strategy for older people.* Dublin: Department of Health; 1998.

11 Moloney O. *Evaluation of the Music in Healthcare Project 2000–2004,* op. cit. p. 24.

12 *Cork Examiner* Christmas at the Lunatic Asylum. December 1876. (Exact date unknown).

13 White M. *An Evaluation of the Cork Mental Health Arts Programme Music Initiative.* Durham: University of Durham (CAHHM); 2008.

14 National Economic and Social Forum. *Mental Health and Social Inclusion: NESF report 36.* Dublin: National Economic and Social Forum; 2007. p. 151.

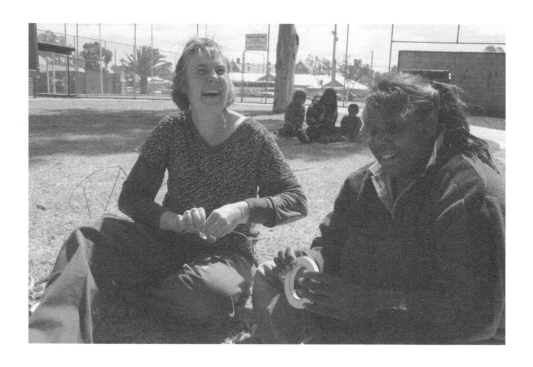

Alison Jones and Catherine Howard making lanterns for the 'Rock Hole Long Pipe' project produced by Community Arts Network WA. PHOTO COURTESY OF POPPY VAN OORDE-GRAINGER

# The preference of the wave: case examples from Western Australia

Australia is still, for us, not a country but a state – or states – of mind. We do not yet speak from within her, but from outside: from the state of mind that describes, rather than expresses, its surroundings, or from the state of mind that imposes itself upon, rather than lives through, landscape and event.

Judith Wright, *The Upside Down Hut*[1]

There is a protocol amongst surfers that the furthest out or longest waiting gets the preference of the wave. If that maxim were applied metaphorically to those who have at one time been socially excluded but are now drawn into community through arts activity, it would appear that creative expression can crest a wave of social change.

We are currently seeing a transformation of community art from confrontational preoccupations with class culture to empathic techniques of social engagement that can simultaneously identify and address need in disadvantaged communities. The ethos of community art now underpins the emergence of joined-up government, enlightened enterprise and a new civil society in which the economics of well-being is a key determinant of policy. The seminal influence in Australia of John Hawkes' *The Fourth Pillar of Sustainability* has affirmed for many there who are working in socioeconomic regeneration that public participation in cultural activities is the basis of both the creative city and the resilient rural community.[2] Central to this is how a healthy community is sustained by a sense of identity and place.

In a report by the Globalism Institute[3] that assesses the importance of identity and place in community cultural development programmes in Australia that are addressing health issues, I came across the opening quote for this chapter. This certainly spoke to my own disorientation as a temporary visitor to Western Australia (WA), bluffing as a 'foreign expert', but I did not see that such existential dislocation was borne out in community arts practice there; on the contrary, it was often in the artworks produced by 'marginalised' people that the most lucid expressions of identity and place were to be found, helping to orientate me in a strange and wonderful country.

In health promotion we often resort to the metaphor of the journey. We speak of 'mapping' local health needs and providing 'signposting' for people in poor health to access medical services. We talk of treatment 'pathways' and the 'road to recovery'. Such use of metaphor reveals a cultural base to healthcare services, and this may enable us to discern what makes for human flourishing. It illuminates what Ivan Illich termed 'adaptation' in his seminal critique of modern healthcare systems in *Limits To Medicine*,[4] and I can see this as having a spiritual resonance in older Australian culture. When I visited the gold rush town of Kalgoorlie, I met with some indigenous people who told me the story of an Aboriginal elder who, unused to motor travel but in need of medical attention, was driven by a ranger to the nearest clinic, some 200 kilometres away. On arriving there, the old man refused to get out of the vehicle. When asked why, he replied that his spirit was following behind on foot and he must wait for it. It would join him in a few days. This tale, told to me in the crucible of Western Australia, reaffirmed for me that a person's cultural perception of what makes for health is key to shaping a holistic understanding of appropriate treatment and care.

## HEALTHWAY

Healthway was established under the state's Tobacco Control Act 1990 and came to life in February 1991. It is a health promotion foundation, and its primary objective is to improve health in WA. Section 26(8) of the Act states that at least 15% of Healthway money is to go to the arts. Healthway looks for sponsorship opportunities through which it can demonstrate long-term health promotion and community benefits, artistic development and the increased involvement and participation of its target priority groups. The sponsorship programme has an annual total budget of AUS$18 million, and about $3 million of that is available for arts sponsorship. That amounts to something not far short of what Arts Council England spends on arts in health in a year. In terms of its regional focus, Healthway directs around $600 000 (23%) of arts sponsorship funds specifically to support arts projects and initiatives in rural and remote communities. It also runs a programme called Aussie Optimism, which is focused in schools and is something similar to the Healthy Schools Standard work in the UK.

In Healthway's *Health Priorities Review 2007*,[5] the current five priority areas were mental health (priority health issue), aboriginal people (priority population), poor nutrition, physical inactivity and smoking (priority risk factors). Ten per cent of arts funding goes on indigenous projects and 60% on young people, which suggests more tracking evaluation is needed. Healthway's strategy report for 2004–07 asserted that its intervention in providing health sponsorship for arts and sports events had had a significant impact in lowering tobacco consumption in the state and had impacted on other areas of health lifestyle.[6] Activity has tended, however, to be focused on raising health awareness through identification with arts and sports events rather than through engagement with specific communities. Healthway has only just begun to support work from the ground up in the development of new traditions within communities (particularly rural and indigenous communities) that can address health issues – but it does want to move into that kind of intervention.

Smoking cessation has been reiterated as the prime focus for Healthway for the next triennium. I wondered if the issue got too much attention, given that the social tide has turned, legislation is in place and cessation is easier to measure. More attention is arguably required now on intersectoral working to address obesity and inactivity, which equally affect indigenous and excluded or poor communities, and on the hidden 'epidemic' of mental ill health. I was surprised to discover that there is no community mental health service in WA (unlike in the UK), only clinical psychology.

The *Health Priorities Review* considers that the delivery on Healthway's mental health priority has been weak, except in the research area, where there are indications that there are ancillary mental health benefits from all kinds of participation. It also argues that more attention should be given to work with elders in future, as the current demographic of beneficiaries is heavily youth-targeted. The review argues that Healthway should henceforth deploy its functions of providing sponsorship grants, scholarships and research in conjunction rather than in separate silos and thereby support team-based, research-guided practice.

Healthway has a proven track record of success in disseminating health education effectively to a vastly dispersed population, but consequently it has not risked changing its approach to meet new challenges, unlike VicHealth, the state health promotion agency for Victoria that also supports the arts. It is worth comparing the two organisations whilst recognising that there is no UK equivalent to either of them.

## VICHEALTH, VICTORIA

VicHealth and Healthway started around the same time, with the abolition of tobacco sponsorship in the early 1990s, but by 2000 VicHealth had changed direction and started to look more at social indicators of health and well-being, particularly via mental health work. Therefore it changed its arts approach and encouraged proposals for developing participation models in arts in community health, rather than straightforward sponsorship.

Perth (in WA), I learned, is more conservative than Melbourne, and Victoria is very much a dynamic state. It has a strong culture-led approach in the state government. VicHealth's budget is about AU$2 million for arts per annum and so is slightly less than that of Healthway. It is an independent statutory body under the Minister for Health, but it has bipartisan support, and there are representatives from different political parties on its board. It will co-fund activities with the state government, as well as fund autonomously when it simply thinks a project is worthy of support. VicHealth has a mental health and well-being course that is used to induct cross-sector workers into arts and health work, similar to Common Knowledge though not as fully developed in its ideas and application. The course supports the development of project planning and evaluation skills, and encourages the research agenda to focus very much on capacity-building. There is little schools-based work, however, in VicHealth's work, largely because it does not want to be drawn into the education system, fearing it would simply dilute strengths too quickly.

A VicHealth video called *Creative Connections*[7] convinced me in 10 minutes there was little I could say to the arts in health sector in the state that they did not already know from experience. There are so many correspondences between arts approaches to community health in Victoria and the practice as I understand it in the UK. On the video, community arts organisation Westside Circus talks about there being a family feeling to its work that provides a catalyst for creating a new community. This organisation focuses on empowering young people through building both physical strength and relationships. Other groups featured on the video include an arts and disability project called Club Wild, similar to the learning-difficulties-sector arts groups the Lawnmowers and Heart n Soul in the UK; and Torch, an issue-based theatre group that works with indigenous communities and sees drama as a way to get conversation going around locally specific health and social issues. VicHealth helps organise projects like these into a forum and network to support sustainability and autonomy.

A momentum for arts in community health has clearly developed through VicHealth, and although it is the agencies it has supported that have taken the work forward, VicHealth really is a powerful facilitator. VicHealth refines its programme about every three years, but mental health is a continuing priority.[8] There is a sense of urgency to the development of this work, and the voluntary sector is very involved, approaching the issue from a social justice agenda. There are, however, almost no studio-based arts activities for mental health service clients like those found in the UK; an exception is the Artful Dodgers' Studio, which has been set up by artists and is run with Jesuit Social Services. Clients at the Artful Dodgers' Studio have dual diagnoses (addiction and mental ill health) and are offered a phased development programme in arts that has a horizontal process, building trust, creativity and capacity, combined with a vertical process, taking clients into purposeful creativity towards group exhibition, the ultimate aim being to redirect them into education and employment. This is seen as long-term work, as the clients progress in two- to three-year cycles, but funding is too short-term for this, so there is a discontinuity in an otherwise exemplary arts project trying to achieve social aims.[9]

With a growing environmental perspective on health, VicHealth has helped initiate arts projects that work with Melbourne's transport system, focusing on train stations as creative community hubs. A development plan was produced in 2007 that has brought key players in the transport sector together, headed by the Department of Infrastructure, which has overall responsibility for transport.[10] With a concern to foster a sense of identity and place, the initiative's advisory committee has linked up with Neighbourhood Renewal and other regeneration schemes, because one of the key aims is to change the appearance and improve the safety of a large number of unstaffed stations in the suburbs. The enthusiasm of both private and public-sector interests in the transport system is really driving this forward, and there are nine local councils signed up to participate in the programme, with an eventual goal of spanning the entire city and suburbs.

VicHealth is able to cross-reference support from all its functions, so the arts in health programme is not pursued in isolation but can draw in all the other aspects of the organisation's work to support it, covering a wide gambit of health promotion. VicHealth believes that no one else is doing it this way in Australia, and a 'hybrid worker' approach is increasingly seen as the way forward in arts in community health. Like Healthway, VicHealth gives a framework for funded projects to work to, and the dissemination of the learning from those projects is crucial. It has also assisted the development of an evaluation toolkit for community-based arts in health projects.[11]

## A CHALLENGE FOR AUSTRALIA

Although I consider VicHealth to be at the forefront of practice internationally, it is Healthway that addresses the greater challenge, a challenge that transcends already difficult population health issues and lies uncomfortably at the core of Australian society; namely the welfare and prospects of indigenous people. On 13 February 2008, newly incumbent Prime Minister Kevin Rudd delivered a historic apology to indigenous people, pledging to 'close the gap that lies between us in life expectancy, educational achievement and economic opportunity.'[12]

The question of how the social inclusion issues that underpin a health crisis in the indigenous population can be tackled with cultural sensitivity places the practice of arts in health in Western Australia at the forefront of socially engaged arts and education. There could be benefit to practitioners internationally in learning from the experience of Healthway and the arts initiatives that it supports in this unique demographic.

Healthway's 2007 priorities review advocates a policy on indigenous people's health that is driven by recognition of social determinants of health, with less emphasis than previously on an individualised cognitive-change approach. There is also a shift to paying more attention to the right settings in which to get engagement – the 'congenial space' factor – and to developing relationships.

The indigenous peoples in WA are in a dire situation; their health profile is such that they commonly live up to 17 years less than people in more affluent urban communities. So there is huge disparity in health and equality, and the health profile of indigenous people is aggravated further by the difficulty in obtaining fresh fruit and vegetables and by generally poor diet and damaging levels of alcohol, drug and solvent usage. To engage effectively with indigenous communities, Healthway has come to recognise that there is a need to move away from health-sector targets in the short term, with the view to affecting community health in the longer term. This could link imaginatively with the cultural planning strategies in local authorities.

Furthermore, the new Public Health Act in Australia provides local government from 2008 with the option to develop public health and community well-being, and Healthway's review argues this is a means to get more effective partnership working in local government settings. However, I noted in one international comparative table in the review[13] that 'capacity-building' is only seen as a strategic priority in the UK. It states that sustainability in a health promotion perspective requires attention to an intervention's effects rather than the means to deliver them – but surely the working relationships developed through capacity-building are essential to maintain a joined-up vision that underpins sustainability?

The State Government Community Development and Justice Standing Committee report *Impact of the Arts in Regional Western Australia*[14] is illuminating on the motivation for local arts development, which is akin to the participation models of local authorities in the UK but with some distinct emphases. The report recognises that arts produce health outcomes and that too much responsibility is placed on volunteers – the main recommendation is for regional arts development officers. The arts are non-competitive, and that is felt to be of value in this sports-obsessed society. Local arts encourage a sense of place to prevent migration to cities and animate small towns as viable alternatives. This is seen as key to having surviving in-place communities, as opposed to the 'fly-in fly-out' communities created by contract workers in the mining industries.

The *Impact of the Arts* report cites several interesting health-focused projects, such as a child health service in Kalgoorlie that started out as an artist residency and the Buyu project, where it was necessary to understand that Aborigines have a different cultural interpretation of 'smoking', because 'when indigenous people thought of smoking they thought of smoke as part of a healing ceremony.' The health professional attached to this project, paediatrician Dr Christine Jeffries-Stokes, saw the need for T-shirts that distinguished between 'good' and 'bad' smoke, and these have been distributed throughout the desert. Healthway funded the Aboriginal art group Wongutha Birni to lead on this. The report was not subsequently taken up by the state government, however; it simply 'informs'. In particular, arts development with indigenous communities is linked with a raft of socioeconomic and health issues, and a specific recommendation is for an inquiry into indigenous arts to be established with the brief to examine matters such as their effect on health, well-being, recidivism and literacy, and to look also at copyright and marketing issues.

## COMPARING PRACTICE

In comparing arts in health practice in northern England and Western Australia, it seems that, unlike the situation with our American cousins, we do speak the same language, but the 'intonation' behind the work is decidedly different. It would be impossible to apply the observation of Judith Wright, quoted at the beginning of this chapter, to northern England. That region's landscape is overcrowded with meaning, and while some rural areas appear unchanged, the towns and cities have been totally transformed by multiculturalism and the transition to a post-industrial era that has left a legacy of health inequalities. The health 'black spots', for example, exactly match the contours of the former coalfield areas. Here, within a new social underclass riddled with the consumer diseases of our time, there is a sense of dislocation borne of economic change rather than geography, but the common ground with Australia is that this dislocation's impact on health is chronically experienced as social exclusion. Arts interventions addressing community mental health go to the heart of the social exclusion problem, and they may also inform the use of arts to address other health promotion issues.

My advance reading of documents from Healthway and other regional arts agencies had suggested to me that I would find a similarity in approach to community-based arts in health in WA. Instead I found a series of fairground mirrors presenting enlarged or diminutive reflections of the characteristics of practice I know from the UK. Basic assumptions I had made about practice in WA have been overturned. Firstly, arts in community health is not clearly defined as an area of informed practice relevant to a wide gamut of social and educational policy; it seems to be regarded more as an effect of cultural planning generating individual and social well-being. Secondly, there are strange bedfellows that sometimes use unfamiliar terminology; for example, disability arts and arts in mental health seem happily to co-exist under the umbrella of social inclusion work in an organisation like DADAA, whereas in the UK they would have to be ideologically separated at birth. This may be because health and well-being are constantly linked in Australia, so there is less friction over drawing connections between disability arts and health. Thirdly, the evidence base from arts agencies in WA for the health benefits of participation in creative activities is slim, despite them being grounded in evaluation theory and reflective practice. Healthway, on the other hand, has consistently provided sound quantitative evidence of the effectiveness of health messaging at arts events, but it has not so far engaged in longitudinal qualitative research to examine how arts engagement might strengthen social determinants of health.

The next difference, with the significant exception of DADAA, whose work I shall describe later, is that there is much less on-the-ground dialogue and opportune partnership-making between the arts sector and health/medical services than I had anticipated; perhaps, ironically, due in part to Healthway's success in sustaining substantial grant resources and logistical support for health-promoting arts events. The most helpful overturned assumption is realising that work patterns in arts in health are not fixed in WA, so adaptable models are evolving, and everything is up for expansive change in an accelerated economy with a participation ethos that seems refreshingly uncynical – in short, having the best New World values – and the well-being of indigenous peoples appears to be at the heart of everyone's concern for ethical practice.

My broad impression of community-based arts and health practice in WA and northern England is this: we have similar ideological practice and aims but view things from opposite ends of the telescope. The Healthway model in WA is focused on effective health messaging that is branded to events, with long experience in this approach enabling it to implement social marketing techniques that would be the envy of health promotion services in the UK. Its research has been largely concerned with assessing message awareness based on quantitative survey methods. The arts sector has partnered with Healthway under a sponsorship model that assists the delivery of cultural product, but, aside from some developmental grant schemes that support cultural planning, there has been little sense of making joint inquiry into the health of specific communities and how that might be improved through long-term arts engagement. Everything disseminates to the big picture of a healthy WA. Any statewide strategic development of arts in health is hampered by a lack of sub-regional arts coordinators, despite this being strongly advocated in the state government report I refer to above and in Regional Arts Australia's *National Directions* report.[15] In northern England, conversely, the focus has been more on developing supportive community contexts for the creative expression of health awareness, sustained through dedicated facilities for arts in health or through multi-sector networks that nurture social integration through creative activities. The research focus is more on qualitative ethnographic study. Everything gravitates to specific at-risk communities reconnecting to health through culture.

The biggest difference, with ultimate relevance to identity and place, lies in mind-boggling geography. In the UK, urban and rural areas sit cheek-by-jowl, so although there are moderations in health needs and how they are addressed, there is still a basic equity in health services. Physical isolation, however acutely felt on a psychological level, may in reality be little more than the infrequency of a rural bus service. WA, on the other hand, is largely composed of wilderness and desert the size of northern Europe and Scandinavia, with most of its two million population concentrated in a hundred-mile coastal strip around Perth. In the Outback, distance feels almost inter-planetary, and there are places with no discernible horizon – like Lake Ballard, site of sculptor Antony Gormley's sentinel figures, where the vast salt flats dissolve into the shimmer of white-hot air. Amidst this kind of infinity and beyond, how and what health services can be delivered creatively to far-flung communities, apart from preventative health education, is a matter of survival strategy. In Australia everything is dictated by land, and the geographic distances make a big difference to policy and action in WA compared to, say, Victoria, where transport logistics and communications are easier. There is no equitable distribution of resources in the country, and above a basic standard of public services, each state fights for its share.

The State of Western Australia Health Department has dissolved its own health promotion unit and has devolved this function to Healthway, as well as to some voluntary-sector organisations such as cancer and heart foundations. Health promotion remains relatively under-funded, partly because there is little evidence base to help argue for increase. Service provision is divided between Metro Health for the urban areas and Country Health for the rural areas. Low wages and the isolation of rural settlements make job retention difficult – many defect into industry – and there is a looming job crisis in public health. Teleconferencing is increasingly used to connect health staff in remote areas, but most have little programme budget. Occupational therapists do more health and safety work than health promotion, yet obesity, for example, will soon be higher than in the US.[16] There are equivalents to the UK's Healthy Schools coordinators in parts of the state, but they have no evident connection with the arts. WA's education curriculum is felt to be seriously overloaded. It could be a strong pathway for health education, but it is too politically complex at present.

More hopefully, there are precedents for developing new social traditions at the interface of health, education and culture in WA in the long-term projects of arts-sector organisations such as DADAA, Country Arts and Community Arts Network Western Australia (CANWA). There is also the Healthway-sponsored Act-Belong-Commit campaign of Mentally Healthy Western Australia, which takes a whole-community approach with grassroots cultural development, and which mirrors techniques used in the UK's Healthy Living networks and Health Trainers initiatives but applies them to more communally based activities.[17]

## ACT-BELONG-COMMIT (A-B-C)

Curtin University's Health Research Unit ran a two-year (2005–07) pilot programme in community mental health in five small towns, funded by Healthway
with Lotterywest and WA Country Health. Each town had a half-time project
coordinator who developed local cultural and community networks to promote
positive mental health. Each coordinator kept a log to be used as the basis
of a book on the programme. Each project also had a half-time intervention
evaluator paired with the coordinator or combined into a single full-time post.
The focus was on building capacity in small-town communities, consisting of
the goldfields 'boomtown' of Kalgoorlie, the coastal towns of Esperance and
Albany, a remote contractor settlement called Karratha and the wheat-belt town
of Northam.

Northam, serving a settled farming population, saw possibly the most
successful project. Here, the head of recreation services said that A-B-C had
significantly changed his shire council's ways of working, declaring that 'time
invested in partnering is time well-spent.' Local mental health services proved
reluctant to engage with the initiative, however, indicating a gulf between A-B-C's
approach and that of conventional services, although links were strengthened
between other health services and the community, providing a 'one-stop shop'
on a 'healthy living centre' model. The project coordinator pinpointed a key
difficulty with the sponsorship model in that 'the branding of messages implied
activities were driven by a campaign, and not by community groups.'

A-B-C showed that, overall, the arts did not have as strong a take-up rate as
sports, but they did show sufficient potential to merit a follow-up three-year
phase that Country Health and Healthway were keen to support. The urban
Metro Health services were less enthused, perhaps suggesting a more meaningful
partner dialogue is required. The retention of A-B-C's project officers has been
difficult, but the longest-serving will now mentor the next wave. This kind of
programme is not as developed as are the mental health initiatives of VicHealth
in Victoria.

The programme reflects processes and key values of arts in community
health projects, and the Act-Belong-Commit slogan indeed parallels issues of
participation, integration and responsibility. The method of developing the local
networks for this initiative shows some similarity with the Common Knowledge
approach I outlined in Chapter 3, though it is much looser and less focused on
quality and sustained arts intervention; rather, it is just basically getting any and
every local voluntary activity to have a positive mental health dimension.

A-B-C could become a bit simplistic at times, but the amount of volunteering
and connection the campaign has generated suggests strong sustainability. The
initiative presents an opportunity to scale up arts activities into local campaigns.
With A-B-C projects now in their second phase, their local steering committees
are helping sustain many activities set up in the first two years. There has been

growth in local media support, and primary care and public health staff have become increasingly involved. There is still a big emphasis on logo visibility, but Healthway has gone beyond the sponsorship model here in its support for research-guided projects in specific communities over time. Thirty-four other rural areas wanted to be involved in the phase two roll out, suggesting that a peer model relationship could be developed between towns and shire counties.

## CANWA

CANWA (Community Arts Network Western Australia) has been running for 20 years, and since then other specialist community arts agencies in WA such as DADAA and Country Arts have emerged. While there have been successful joint collaborations between agencies, there is some risk of duplication. There is also an unspoken competition for survival, which has been created ironically not by a lack of resources so much as a shift to the entrepreneurial application of the arts to training and community development programmes, where the transformational power of arts has to be played out across a wide gamut of social policy agendas. This could lead to an over-diversification of practice unless countered by a strong sense of mission and a focus on long-term work in specific communities – in CANWA's case, in the goldfield and wheatbelt regions. CANWA's work interestingly aspires to build the practice of arts in health within schools (unusual in WA compared to England) and to develop complementary practice between art therapies and community arts in work with indigenous communities.

All across WA, changes to local political boundaries and the public's resistance to them are further undermining a sense of place and identity. Cultural planning in the shire authorities tends to be seen as creating tourist attractions or as just a form of window-dressing for an Outback boom economy rather than as being about meaningful local development. Value systems and coherence are disappearing, there is no sense of history, and the new affluence of the young is breaking up intergenerational bonds. Indigenous people are particularly disempowered in that respect. Indigenous arts are growing but more for small-scale enterprise than for revitalising community. Mining is now the powerhouse of the economy again, and while mining companies support local arts development, there is ambiguity in it. A lot of CANWA's work seems to coalesce around these issues, and it is trying to strengthen its voice on them. CANWA's activities offer interesting perspectives on issues of meaning around identity and place in WA. Its work is highly relevant to public health and mental health issues and to the social integration advocated in Premier Rudd's apology to indigenous peoples following the 2007 election.

CANWA focuses on targeting state and local government funds and Healthway sponsorship, and its activities comprise cultural mapping and planning, grant-giving to local voluntary groups and training in arts management, with an underlying ethos of promoting well-being and social justice. These functions can overlap; for example, its Community Culture fund covers both cultural mapping and planning. Mapping involves grassroots consultation to determine what provision local people would like, and planning is a cultural strategy driven by local authority support and usually involving a consultant in its formulation.

CANWA's practice is well grounded in international thinking on social inclusion and social capital. Its research agenda,[18] and particularly its work on youth inclusion,[19] clearly grasp what I believe is most crucial in arts in community health work: an awareness of how to evolve relationship-based work through network development. CANWA is concerned that Healthway does not sufficiently understand or support cultural planning, focusing on settings for delivery (with lots of logo promotion) rather than network relationships and planning.

CANWA has both proactive and responsive grant functions – and I am not sure there is any UK equivalent of this, except in some local authorities' arts services. It provides advice on applications to other funders and assists capacity-building. It undertakes occasional big projects that aim for sustainability; there is currently one in the goldfields on public art and one in the wheatbelt on storytelling. Big projects are inevitably viewed as showcases of what the whole organisation is about, but the development of these two projects at first seemed to me to be tangential and limited to an 'outreach' model; they should rather be treated as 'a perfect pair' and have the back-up administration and on-the-ground support that their other showcase project in Kellerberrin has enjoyed. The timetable for these projects was so tight that the sustainability issue had to be addressed from the outset.

Kellerberrin, a wheatbelt town 150 miles east of Perth, was chosen in 2006 for a long-term CANWA project because it offered potential for a vibrant indigenous culture, despite socioeconomic hardship. It is an established site for a traditional Aboriginal corroboree (a ceremonial meeting) and for the Keela Dreaming Festival, which includes dance, song and storytelling. CANWA also recognised the need to address the stress affecting the white community. Farmers in the wheatbelt are being forced out of farming because of prolonged drought, and this crisis is further aggravated by young people in rural communities preferring moving to the city to carrying on the family tradition of farming.

Two years into the project, Kellerberrin aspired to have an Aboriginal cultural centre and a gallery showcasing both white and Aboriginal contemporary art as part of a town redevelopment plan. The indigenous Noongar people want this. A women's group now leads CANWA's arts and crafts development, and the 'community mob' leaders are women. Visual art is highly appreciated, though young men are difficult to involve, especially if the session artists are women. There are also 'avoidance relationships' to be aware of; these are often based on cultural taboos. Another aspiration is to have a Noongar language centre, and the Noongar women have requested art therapy as part of counselling services. The introduction of communal eating into events at Kellerberrin has proved a simple but effective way of bringing individual projects together. Such cross-currents really sparkle in CANWA's programme; generally I get the sense of its work being based in real emergent community rather than in the art world.

CANWA is adept at inviting key staff in state government departments to visit Kellerberrin. The town is clearly a testing ground for long-term cultural development work with an indigenous community, and the support evident for the project on the part of key decision-makers in the state government shows it is seen as a development model.

The deployment of indigenous arts staff, plus the combination of the old (in the traditional corroboree and the Keela Dreaming Festival) and the new (in the aspiration for a cultural and language centre) gives it a strong base. The success of an annual town hall ball for the indigenous community is an early indicator of how well embedded the project has become in establishing new traditions. The Noongar women's interest in having art therapy as part of a counselling service suggests they grasp the connection between participatory arts and well-being, and the combination of art therapy and arts in community health would make for interesting exploration of joint practice.

Police in Kellerberrin have noticed a reduction in call-outs to incidents in the indigenous community, and young women are noticeably drinking less when a workshop programme is running. This community has in the past had a strong Methodist religion, but elders are concerned that the adult generation has now become dysfunctional. This dysfunction is largely due to alcoholism and the painful unspoken legacy of the 'stolen generation', when Aborigine children were forcibly removed to foster homes under eugenics-influenced policies. There have been occasional clashes between animist religious beliefs in spirits of the land and Christian orthodoxy, but it is the songs of Methodism that have tended to sustain the community through dark times.

A Healthway grant scheme titled Sharing Stories, which CANWA administers, could have an important role in revitalising indigenous storytelling. It has only a short history, with a handful of grant applications, and it needs a better dynamic – the projects described in the booklet are great, however, and this fund has real potential. It could work across other CANWA initiatives.[20] Sharing Stories offers opportunities for intergenerational work, which is at the core of arts and health work because it can deliver in social integration. As a CANWA staff member observed, it is 'a grant where you can get a lot out of a process', and understanding that process is vital if we are to better validate well-being outcomes.

Health aims are implicit too in CANWA's youth arts work, though the main purpose is to motivate clients back into education or employment. Closer links with health services on this would help to validate its well-being outcomes. CANWA's Perth-based youth programme Fired Up provides pre-vocational training to teenagers deemed 'unteachable' and has already expanded to seven project bases. The demands of working with this target group mean that staff require support to cope with the emotional difficulties presented to them, but, just as in the UK, there are no funds for this. I suspect youth arts is in the frontline of the mental health service in Perth by default, because suicide is the biggest cause of death in under-25s.

## COUNTRY ARTS WA

Country Arts WA covers regional touring but also focuses on local arts development. There is functionally some overlap with CANWA, though Country Arts does not do cultural planning work. Most of its staff are funded through contract work from the Department of Culture and Arts in the state government. Generally arts work is low paid, however, and the boom economy is impacting on staff retention.

Country Arts' Out There programme undertakes youth arts development with specific communities for one year. Its 2007 programme was at Yilii (population 250) near Hall's Creek in the Kimberley. Yilii has one small clinic, and the nearest hospital is in Broome or Derby, over a day's drive away. In 2007 Yilii was being targeted by police to stamp out child abuse. The rates of alcoholism and crime-related violence here are high, and there is peer pressure on young men to drink heavily in nearby towns. Prison is a weak deterrent, often viewed as a holiday offering better living conditions and food. Aborigines constitute 40% of the jail inmates, yet only 3% of the population.

There are no mental health services in this part of the Kimberley, and there seems to be a general demoralisation in health workers. Indigenous people's non-compliance in their care plans, particularly in diabetes management, is a big issue. Although elsewhere in WA the exploration of fundamental connections between culture and health in indigenous communities has shown potential to realise groundbreaking work, such as the Wanti Sugarba diabetes project that was developed by Dr Jeffries-Stokes,[21] health workers in the Kimberley have been uninterested in the arts, possibly feeling it would just add to their high workload. Yet generic medical services to Aborigines have proved ineffective, and arts workers argue that a special kind of culturally sensitive health service is required.

There are poor education prospects for young people in the Kimberley, and truancy is rife. Tertiary education is almost a non-starter because it would require living away from home, which is antithetical to the culture. Lack of education means the mining industry is not employing Outback indigenous people in significant numbers, despite their land rights. Corporate responsibility is otherwise channelled into community funds that are small relative to the profits.

A huge issue in indigenous communities is how to pass on traditional knowledge of the elders through contemporary media that youth want to explore. So in Yilii, Country Arts invited expressions of interest in a programme with an intergenerational aim. The project involved song-writing workshops, with a 'custodian' elder passing on tribal wisdom to the youth through songs. This was funded through Healthway's Y Culture grant stream for drug awareness. Logo accreditation was required as usual, though Country Arts felt the message had little impact on the general population. However, the young participants were drinking less when in the workshop programme. They now have a touring band known as the Walkabout Boys. The Kimberley is traditionally strong on music, yet eclectic and modern in its taste. After the year's development programme, Country Arts provided follow-up workshops on practical issues like equipment maintenance. Clearly the programme is limited by what can be achieved in just one year.

The need for longer arts engagement with specific communities was reinforced for me when I met Megan Lewis, a photographer who had just completed a five-year self-funded residency with the indigenous community in the Western Desert. She compiled a book of her photos, *Conversations with the Mob*, published in 2008.[22] She also arranged for a selection of the photographs to tour WA with Healthway's support and to have Aborigine health workers on hand to explain the project and to raise health awareness and dietary management in communities by interpreting the exhibition to both indigenous and white audiences. I thought that would be a simple and direct way of connecting health and cultural sectors. She told me the photos would be interspersed with stories and quotes that aimed to capture the cultural identity of the subjects.

Megan Lewis talked about 'walking alongside' the community in a pedagogic role and how it took six months to be able to take a 'true' photo. When she began her residency, she wanted to photograph funerals and was initially refused. She explained that she felt it was important to reflect their emotional life in order to counter prejudice; for example, the trauma of high family fatalities is a compounding factor in why Aborigines find reasons for getting drunk in town. She also encouraged young men to discuss their feelings and identity, particularly because communication with tribal elders about their feelings is difficult and because there are mental health issues for disaffected youth that sometimes result in psychotic episodes. When I suggested that her insight in this community into how feelings are suppressed and given no credence only reflects back our own dysfunctionality, she said that was exactly it; they presented life in the raw, our common humanity and common problems.

The poor diet of indigenous people is not due to supply-chain difficulties but to lack of motivation on the part of white traders. Ironically, expensive drugs can be imported into the Kimberley but not fresh fruit and vegetables. Indigenous people are caught, or rather displaced, between old and new Aboriginal culture and the hegemonic culture of modern Australia and its consumerist front. Megan Lewis made an extraordinary commitment to this project, and the living conditions she endured affected her own health. She also affirmed that health staff in the outback either accept the limitations of medicine or remain in a bubble of applying the culturally insensitive procedures that they have been medically trained in.

## DADAA

DADAA, which stands for Disability in the Arts, Disadvantage in the Arts Australia, was established in 1993 and has developed from a specialist disability arts agency to an organisation with a wider arts in health focus. Originally it worked to a festivals model, with self-advocacy for disabled people as a goal. In recent years, however, DADAA has developed exceptional partnering skills with public, voluntary and corporate sectors, creating a hybrid form of arts development that is so embedded in new models of social engagement, capacity-building and health reform that it is no longer reliant on the arts funding system for its sustainability. Its partnership model now realises a AU$2 million turnover, and service level agreements mean that state and federal policies increasingly inform its work.

DADAA specializes in piloting models; for example, it recently completed a six-year project in Albany to make disability visible through the arts.[23] DADAA currently has long-term field projects evolving with the indigenous community in the Kimberley and in day centres in Bunbury. Each programme has a reference group for participant governance. DADAA takes only an advisory role on these, believing that trust is essential and that quality is determined by debate and the selection of the right artists.

In conjunction with Country Arts WA, DADAA is also at least partially redressing an infrastructural weakness in the state by deploying specialist regional officers in arts and disability. DADAA is more interested in working in public spaces than in institutions, and it stresses the importance of fostering autonomy and self-esteem. In indigenous communities, it works more invisibly through local agencies. Reflective practice is the norm in its team-management approach, and a log is kept of all work, with stringent reporting requirements that are open to participant feedback. International links have been forged with Kenya on mentoring, Hong Kong on training and Ireland (Kilkenny) on performance projects.

Mental health now comprises around half of DADAA's work, mostly funded by federal government services. This community-based work addresses social isolation issues and severe mental illness, and it works with middle managers on service development. Working from taster sessions, longer-term programmes with outcome goals are then devised. DADAA's arts interventions take a non-instrumental approach while maintaining strong referral systems, so it is trusted to say when clinicians should be involved. Its home-base gallery of Freight (in Fremantle) provides studio facilities and arts training for clients, while nurturing a mental health culture. Freight is not hampered by bureaucracy and can focus on practice. DADAA now has a huge informal referral base from psychiatric services, and clinicians initially visit Freight and other DADAA field projects with their clients to help them settle in. DADAA has fixed funding available under service level agreements to offer places, and therefore there are no financial barriers. Pathways are laid into further education, volunteering and jobs, though DADAA also takes readmissions. Community arts and mental health was the subject of the second volume of DADAA's *Disseminate* publications series.[24]

A long-term film project titled *Lost Generation* exemplifies DADAA's approach in being sensitive to the individual need and character of marginalised individuals while having a cumulative power to give voice to an excluded community. *Lost Generation* refers to a group of people with what are termed 'intellectual disabilities' who have been institutionalised for most of their lives and have little or no connection to their community.

The *Lost Generation* project is a four-year partnership between DADAA and the Disability Services Commission's Accommodation Services Directorate, who are able to ensure the ethical integrity of the film-making process on account of their long-standing connections with clients' families and carers. Copyright is retained by the film's subject. The evaluation aims to track the more intangible qualities and outcomes, investigating the impact on families and any improvement in social interaction as a result of seeing the film. The goals are to develop the partnership through tangible resources, to develop relationships between staff and partners in order to support individuals to achieve their aspirations as citizens in their community, and to work with local government to support inclusion.

The project works in 6–9-month cycles, with up to 50 clients in a local government area. *Lost Generation* started as a number of little projects building to a long-term culmination, with each wave of new films being premiered in a local cinema. The project will eventually consist of over 600 short films presenting personal cameos of people with special needs, and DADAA is building an archive through this work. Some of the films are charming vignettes, but others are sharply observed reminders of the real person behind the 'client'. They are increasingly being used in staff training.

DADAA has helped the Disability Services Commission (DSC) to tap into other non-government funds and open a link with the corporate sector. DSC feels that partnership with the arts sector has given expression to its aim to foster well-being by looking at what makes for healthy living within a community care plan. This has been easier to evaluate in a qualitative approach, though a quantitative assessment is also made of health service readmissions. WA has the lowest rate in Australia of institutionalised people, as policy has shifted to providing group homes in the community. DSC's clients, however, often do not have voting rights, so awareness-raising is needed to develop local councillors' knowledge of disenfranchised disabled people. Family empowerment is also crucial to enable relatives, who provide a valued voluntary resource, to act on behalf of their loved one.

Each *Lost Generation* film aims to capture the essence of the subject in order to help the carer to see who that person is. Though it cannot yet prove it, it is thought in DSC that improving connectivity in this way reduces the resource burden for support. It can also demystify disability, with the films providing 'first contact' for excluded people through raising a topic of conversation. DSC believes there is nothing similar going on internationally, and it is looking to get ministerial interest across the states and to exploit the training potential in how this creative approach cuts across portfolios. This is the bigger picture in which DADAA, along with other voluntary-sector agencies, now plays a part. A common goal is for local government to recognise a need for capacity-building to embed new approaches, and agencies sense they are on the cusp of achieving this as local government becomes more proactive.

The dissemination of DADAA's work is now moving into research publications with sponsorship from the mining company Rio Tinto, with whom it enjoys a long-term working relationship. Soon after DADAA first approached Rio Tinto in 2002, its arts development programme in a mining area in the Kimberley faltered due to misunderstandings with the local indigenous community over accountability and ownership. To its credit, Rio Tinto supported DADAA through a difficult and demoralising episode, helping them absorb the learning that has made DADAA a more resilient and sensitively entrepreneurial organisation in the long term. The company felt that DADAA had an innovative community development model to offer, but it needed help to articulate its benefits and make 'good sense' partnership proposals. DADAA's director was subsequently sponsored for a high-level training programme in project management and enterprise.

The Rio Tinto WA Future Fund, established in 2001, takes a partnership approach to corporate giving, with the aim of changing how organisations work in community. The fund has company top-fliers and community representatives on its board. It is supporting inquiry into what creates well-being, and its board grasps the seriousness of the need to get to grips with this issue.

In Rio Tinto sites in WA, over half the population is indigenous, and providing employment preference for this group means it has to tackle all the issues that these disadvantaged communities face. Health is clearly a crucial issue, and Rio Tinto sees a good model for addressing this in recent child health work in the state, although there is some perception that government is not doing enough on local infrastructure development. The 'fly in, fly out' culture of shift working has become a big issue for mining companies, as it impacts on occupational health, family cohesion and industrial relations, both internally and externally. The Rio Tinto WA Future Fund board is concerned that local identity is being lost in the mining towns, as is the pioneer ethic of 'make your own culture'. It therefore looks to DADAA to collect the data and persuasive case studies that offer concrete examples of how a community can shape its identity and be inclusive and sustained. Rio Tinto expects a shift in emphasis in its relationship with DADAA towards the communication of outcomes through publications and replicable models of practice. Along with Healthway, it jointly supports the development of DADAA's *Disseminate* publication series.

With its expansive portfolio and an incremental increase in turnover, DADAA is approaching the level of a major arts production house, and that poses interesting questions, both for the organisation and for its peers in the subsidised arts sector, regarding the quality and value of socially engaged arts. I suspect the challenge for DADAA in future will be how, within its complex web of partnerships, it can move from being the champion of social inclusion possibilities to becoming their actual delivery agent with signed-up partners in the exercise of health for all and social justice. This has similarly tested the mettle of arts-led healthy living centres in the UK in recent years.


## ONLY CONNECT . . .

There are many arts in health projects in northern England that are in parallel with these WA initiatives,[25] and much could be exchanged by way of reciprocal observation, co-mentoring and reflective practice. The CAHHM centre at Durham University and Manchester Metropolitan University's Arts for Health unit are increasingly and proactively involved in developing practice and research in local projects into cluster programmes. Key to the cluster approach is the sharing of meanings around identity and place, and a concern that effective evaluation is developed primarily with and for the participants, not for the funding agencies. This can produce local and individually specific articulations of well-being, and it can also produce a mythology around the arts activities that grounds imaginative perceptions of community – what Australian political commentator Donald Horne has marvellously described as 'the sensation of common cause'.[26] This will help our understanding of how empowerment and social inclusion outcomes, anchored in contextual reflection on identity and place, can be identified and measured. The 'common cause' is what community-based arts in health should now explore and share, so this is the right time to develop international exchange in this field.

What perhaps hinders progress in developing meaningful connections in practice between Australia and the UK is that in Australia the information network for this work is not very good. There was, for a brief time, an artist-led national network, but this folded in 2004.[27] A newly formed organisation called Arts and Health Australia is aiming to re-instate a national network informed by international best practice and high quality research and holds its inaugural conference in November 2009.[28] Not every state has an initiative like Healthway in Western Australia or VicHealth in Victoria, and practitioners in arts in health in the other states feel that the work is sporadic and poorly supported. The Australia Council for the Arts closed down its community development unit in 2004, which severely impacted on arts in health, and there does seem to be widespread dissatisfaction among community arts organisations that the Australia Council is not really grasping the potential that is there and looking at how it could be developed.

The Australia Council for the Arts attempted to re-engage with the field in 2006 by commissioning a strategy option paper produced by the University of Melbourne[29] and through earmarking action research funds for designated 'demonstration projects'. Curiously, most of the reports and articles cited in the literature review in this paper were from the UK; the review overlooked interesting and relevant research originating in Victoria's universities and at Flinders University in South Australia. The paper also does not explain the methodology of its research; it would be useful, for example, to know the questions put to practitioners in the field who were invited to contribute to the study. Responses revealed 90% in favour of the need for a conference and demonstration projects, but only 51% cited a need for capacity-building. I have argued elsewhere that it is capacity-building across the different sectors that can produce interesting pilot projects.

In 2007 the Australia Council for the Arts invited tenders for demonstration projects, encouraging consortium arrangements between, say, an arts organisation, a university department, a health agency and local or state government. There was scope for proposing what was termed a 'hybrid model' encompassing projects addressing the therapeutic nature of arts, and there was also scope for proposals more widely addressing the social inclusion agenda. It was specified in the tender document, however, that the Australia Council wanted to see proposals following a quasi-experimental research design with a control group, thereby limiting the type of project that could be conducted and the type of context in which it would work. It appeared that the Australia Council was directing the initiative towards a research design fitting a medical evidence model and looking for meaningful quantitative as well as qualitative evidence. This made it a challenging scheme, but not one that at the moment readily connects with the social model of health that is as germane to arts in health practice in Australia as it is in the UK.

I believe practitioners in arts in community health in Australia and the UK have a common interest in exploring how participatory arts can produce individual and communal well-being. The ethos and structure of DADAA's Freight gallery in Fremantle and, say, the similarly constituted Artful Dodgers' studios in Melbourne are mirrored in initiatives such as the START studios in Manchester and the mental health studio network of North East England. What experience seems to be telling us at our respective antipodes is that we need a sustainability of practice that is fuelled by vision as well as funding, and we need longitudinal research into relationship-based ways of working in arts and health. An emphasis on sustaining quality relationships around arts participation not only connects with the basis of social capital, it also draws on social psychology from observation of how arts can transform communities. However, the research base for how these two things coalesce seems fraught and fragile, as I shall explain in Chapter 8.

## REFERENCES

1 Wright J. The upside down hut. In: Barnes J, editor. *The Writer in Australia: a collection of literary documents 1856–1964.* Melbourne: Oxford University Press; 1969. p. 332.

2 Hawkes J. *The Fourth Pillar of Sustainability: culture's essential role in public planning.* Melbourne: Cultural Development Network; 2001.

3 Mulligan M, Humphery K, James P, *et al. Creating Community: celebrations, arts and wellbeing within and across local communities.* Melbourne: Globalism Institute RMIT; 2006.

4 Illich I. *Limits To Medicine.* London: Boyars; 1976.

5 Rosenberg M, Wood L, Mills C, *et al. Healthway Health Priorities Review.* Perth: Health Promotion Evaluation Unit of the University of Western Australia; 2007.

6 Healthway. *Healthway Strategic Plan 2004–07.* Perth: Healthway; 2003.

7 VicHealth. *Creative Connections: a video promoting mental health and wellbeing through the arts* [video]. Melbourne: VicHealth; 2004.

8 McLeod J. *Promoting Mental Health through Accessing the Arts.* Melbourne: VicHealth; 2006.

9 Marsden S, Thiele M. P(ART)icipation: art, dual diagnoses and the Artful Dodgers' Studio. In: Lewis A, Doyle D, editors. *Proving the Practice: evidencing the effects of community arts programs on mental health.* Fremantle: DADAA; 2008. pp. 60–73.

10 Village Well. *Train Stations as Places for Community Wellbeing.* Melbourne: VicHealth; 2006.

11 Effective Change Ltd. *Evaluating Community Arts and Community Wellbeing: an evaluation guide for community arts practitioners.* Melbourne: Arts Victoria; 2002. Available at: www.vichealth.vic.gov.au/~/media/ProgramsandProjects/MentalHealthandWell Being/Publications/Attachments/CAPS%20Express%20Evaluation%20Guide.ashx (accessed 5 January 2009).

12 Rudd's Apology Revealed. *Sydney Morning Herald;* 13 February 2008.

13 Rosenberg, Wood, Mills, *et al., op. cit.* p. 45.

14 Parliament of Western Australia Legislative Assembly's Community Development and Justice Standing Committee. *Impact of the Arts in Regional Western Australia.* Perth: Government Printer; 2005.

15 Regional Arts Australia. *National Directions*. Port Adelaide: Regional Arts Australia; 2006.

16 Baker Heart Research Institute. *Australia's Future 'Fat Bomb': a report on the future consequences of Australia's expanding waistline on cardiovascular disease.* Melbourne: Baker Heart Research Institute; 2008. Available at www.bakeridi.edu.au/Assets/Files/FatBomb_report.pdf (accessed 1 February 2009).

17 Donovan R, James R, Jalleh G, *et al.* Implementing Mental Health Promotion: the Act Belong Commit mentally healthy WA campaign in Western Australia. *Int J Ment Health Promot.* 2006; 8(1): 29–38.

18 Sonn C, Drew N, Kasat P. *Conceptualising Community Cultural Development.* Perth: CANWA; 2002.

19 Ruane S. *Paving Pathways for Youth Inclusion: the contribution of community cultural development.* Perth: CANWA; 2007.

20 Community Arts Network Western Australia. *Sharing Stories: community sponsorship bulletin.* Perth: CANWA; 2006.

21 Jeffries-Stokes C. *Wanti Sugarba: a report of the intervention phase of the North Goldfields kidney health project.* Perth: University of Western Australia; 2007.

22 Lewis M. *Conversations with the Mob.* Perth: University of Western Australia; 2008.

23 Kapetas JT. *Unhiding.* Fremantle: DADAA; 2007.

24 Lewis A, Doyle D. *Proving the Practice: evidencing the effects of community arts programs on mental health.* Fremantle: DADAA; 2008.

25 White M. *Determined to Dialogue: a survey of arts in health in the Northern and Yorkshire regions.* University of Durham: CAHHM; 2002.

26 Horne D. *Some Thoughts on 'Cultural Vitality'.* Perth: Department of Culture and the Arts of the State Government of Western Australia; 2004.

27 Australian Network for Arts and Health (defunct). Information available at: www.ccd.net/about/health.html (accessed 3 January 2009).

28 Arts and Health Australia. Available at: www.artsandhealth.org (accessed 3 January 2009).

29 Joubert L, Dunt D, Kellaher M, *et al. Strategy Options in Arts and Health: prepared for the Australia Council for the Arts.* Melbourne: University of Melbourne; 2007.

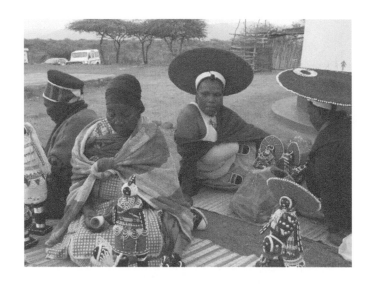

The Siyazama doll-makers. PHOTO: KATE WELLS

# CHAPTER 6

# I am because we are: case examples from South Africa

Land of Joy in Soweto,
Come and join us today
This is colour yellow!
This is colour red!
Colour blue!
Colour green!
Come and join us today!
Keep up the good work and shine!

Soweto children's playground song

Both epidemiology[1] and social capital theory[2] attest that social integration is a key determinant of health. In a newly liberated nation such as South Africa, this tenet may be especially important as both a low-cost spur for improving public health and the buffer for sustaining it in a difficult socioeconomic climate. In southern Africa, sociability connects with a deep-rooted philosophy. The concept of ubuntu, or humanity, finds its expression in proverbs and sayings such as the Sotho maxim 'motho ke motho ka batho' (a person is a person by people) or in the Zulu words 'imuntu ngumuntu ngabantu', meaning that one's humanity is defined through sociability.[3] On the last page of his autobiography, *Long Walk To Freedom*,[4] Nelson Mandela affirms this first principle of ubuntu as the basis for personal and national reconciliation as he generously recognises that the perpetrators of oppression can themselves be 'prisoners' of an iniquitous system.

This humanism underpinning a political struggle has filtered into the proclaimed 'miracle' of South Africa as the saving grace of a troubled nation whose leadership is seen to be falling short on delivering the promise of the post-apartheid era.[5] As President Thabo Mbeki said in his Nelson Mandela Memorial Lecture in July 2006:

> the great masses of our country everyday pray that the new South Africa that is being born will be a good, a moral, a humane and a caring South Africa which as it matures will progressively guarantee the happiness of all its citizens . . . because of the infancy of our brand new society, we have the possibility to act in ways that would, for the foreseeable future, infuse the values of Ubuntu into our very being as a people.[6]

Without tackling a weak economy, soaring crime and the growing number of attacks on refugees, however, such exhortation is unlikely to raise the stock of social capital.

Ubuntu is itself challenged by the social destruction wreaked by modern-day plague. An economic advisor to Johannesburg's city government told me anecdotally that in 2005 in the municipal authorities of South Africa the biggest single item of civic expenditure shifted from water supply to land acquisition – because they needed more cemeteries. South Africa now has the highest prevalence of HIV/AIDS in the world, with almost six million people living with the disease, and half of these are women in heterosexual relationships.[7] In 2002 it had been hoped that the HIV/AIDS virus in South Africa had peaked at an adult infection rate of one in five.[8] In 2005 the South African Department of Health estimated a national infection figure of just under one-third of the adult population. The province of KwaZulu-Natal is the worst hit area; for example, research into HIV-infected pregnant women conducted at Hlabisa Hospital in 2000 projected an infection rate of one in three sexually active people in the region.[9]

There has in the past been prevarication in the South African government's response to the extent of the epidemic, and preventative health strategies have not been based sufficiently on research. There is evidence, for example, that male circumcision may reduce HIV transmission by as much as 60%, but tribal rites of circumcision are now poorly practised.[10] There are calls for a state campaign for male circumcision so that men's health can be at the forefront of the AIDS message. Government policy on HIV/AIDS has sometimes been confused, and Mandela's declaration that 'AIDS is no longer just a disease; it is a human rights issue' has been politically skewed by Mbeki to argue that poverty and unfair trade are the root cause of AIDS.[11] Research has confirmed the need, however, to address AIDS in a broad context, because effective intervention must deal with more than the health disaster; it must transform the related socioeconomic context.[12]

The scale of the epidemic and its implications for the country's already weak human-resource infrastructure helps explain why it appears that every other advertising billboard and every school wall carries an AIDS message. Much of this messaging has been artist-designed, deploying both one-off images and multiples. In addition, there has been a plethora of theatre groups touring drama productions on sexual health to urban and rural areas, and there has been health messaging through mass media interventions such as the work of the Soul City Institute media education agency[13] and the *Tsha Tsha* teenage TV 'soap'. Collectively termed 'edutainment' rather than arts in health, this work has been extensively evaluated.[14] Studies suggest, however, that while these interventions have significantly raised awareness on sexual health issues, they have had limited impact in changing behaviour.

A series of international expert workshops convened by the United Nations' HIV/AIDS programme with Penn State University noted that existing models focus primarily on individual behaviour and make little allowance for the role of the social and environmental context of disease-prevention interventions.[15] It was also observed that the 'edutainment' approach cannot be pursued effectively in isolation; it must be accompanied by an adequate infrastructure for providing services or it will not have strong effects in changing audience behaviour. There is growing recognition that the 'edutainment' intervention lacks models of engagement and also the time and resources to work in-depth with specific target groups. Arts-based intervention has therefore begun to work within community development rather than simply in a health information context.[16]

DramAidE is an arts company based in Durban and formed in 1992. It has attempted to address the HIV/AIDS crisis by combining the mass-messaging approach of touring theatre with more residency-based performance work around life skills targeted at selected schools. The company specialises in theatre for sex education, and its facilitators speak and perform in both English and Zulu. Initially the company just presented original plays for young audiences on HIV/AIDS themes, but in recent years DramAidE has shifted the emphasis from persuasive messaging to what it terms 'information gathering in an ongoing cultural conversation', with the drama provision moving from a didactic to a more empathic and improvisational approach.

The DramAidE website[17] reveals that the organisation has become much more about participatory drama, with programmes that include establishing peer educators in schools, supporting health promoters (who are similar to the health trainers in the UK whom I described in Chapter 2), capacity-building for 'caring communities', and offshoot projects addressing topics such as domestic and in-school violence and hygiene. They also develop vegetable gardens in schools and do candlelight memorials for AIDS victims. An important core technique used is forum theatre, which encourages audiences to instigate role-play and improvisation.

DramAidE's own evaluation of its work has attempted to use a logical framework approach to gather and analyse data (an example of this will be given in Chapter 8). This has the advantage of being able to integrate project planning, internal monitoring and evaluation, but the downside is that some aspects of the intervention are difficult to pin down into single objectives and outcomes. DramAidE's director, Lynn Dalrymple, has noted that:

> The Logical Framework Approach sets goals and targets and its implementation requires top-down management. This leaves very little space for rapid changes of plan if it is seen that the intervention does not meet the needs of the target group. The emphasis on quantitative measures (rather than qualitative inferences or a combination of both) may result in a distorted interpretation of the meanings and realities in observed behaviours.[18]

Adherence to this model has also been frustrated by the complexity inherent in arts in health work in attributing outcome to input. Tackling this may require a longitudinal study perspective, if that can be resourced, as well as more interdisciplinary action research.

Addressing HIV/AIDS through the arts in South Africa has to be understood in the political context of a liberated nation that is still deeply traumatised by its apartheid history. Under apartheid the white community in South Africa produced arts using styles, techniques and materials imported from Europe – ironically at a time when European artists were freely referencing African influences in their work. Western conventions, iconography and (mainly European) history of art formed the curriculum content, and cultural values were taught largely through religious studies. National Christian education as developed by the state and endorsed by most churches lay the foundation for a racially divided society in a Christian state that claimed biblical authority for the superiority of whites. Indigenous arts of the black majority, on the other hand, found expression in a culture of resistance. Art proved a powerful medium for affirming social injustice; as an activist arts teacher told me, 'In Soweto in the 1980s, even exhibitions were arrested.'

Agitprop art, however, can have an inherent weakness. In 1989, near the end of the apartheid era, Albie Sachs, a political activist and victim of a state terrorist murder attempt, addressed some provocative thoughts on culture to his fellow members of the ANC. He argued for a ban on the use of the metaphor of 'culture as a weapon':

> A gun is a gun, and if it were full of contradictions, it would fire in all sorts of directions and be useless for its purpose. Art and literature, on the other hand, deal in ambiguity and complexity. Artists need to explore the world around them in all its complexity, and this includes artists who are members of the liberation movement. However, such a subtle task is not one to which they are accustomed. Instead of getting real criticism, we get solidarity criticism. Our

artists are not pushed to improve the quality of their work; it is enough that it be politically correct.[19]

The new South Africa has one of the most progressive constitutions in the world (which Sachs had a key role in drawing up), leading in human rights, gender equity, protection of minority rights and cultural diversity, and arts and cultural education are constitutionally guaranteed for every child. But while the government has penned the notion of an 'African Renaissance', the vast socioeconomic difficulty facing the country has meant there has been a significant lack of investment in the development of liberal arts and art training, and there has been a lack of support for voluntary arts organisations to undertake constructive partnerships with civil society. The government's alternative use of politically correct mass media as 'spin doctors', such as in the controversial 'loveLife' billboard campaign,[20] has been met with apathy and scorn. As DramAidE's experience suggests, even when there are avenues to linking arts, health and education in the face of population health crisis, it is hard to achieve sustained improvement in a model of social change that must be sensitive to complex tribal cultures as well as to human rights.

## SIYAZAMA

I began this book with a description of a project in South Africa that has been providing long-term community engagement, the Siyazama project in KwaZulu-Natal, which was developed through the Department of Design Studies at Durban University of Technology.[21] Siyazama focuses on two groups: rural craftswomen from Muden in the district of Msinga, 150 miles north of Durban, and women artists (and some men) from an area closer to the city known as The Valley of a Thousand Hills.

Set up by the head of design, Dr Kate Wells, in 1997, Siyazama (roughly translated as 'we are trying') interweaves the health education, life skills and economic development of rural women through the regeneration of traditional bead crafts. It has also become a powerful medium for articulating sexual health issues, sometimes graphically through imagery and tableaux. Wells' ongoing research interest, as expressed in her Ph.D. thesis, has been 'aimed at assessing the value of this type of creative interactive work with rural women, the effectiveness of metaphorical expression through beadwork with regard to sensitive issues, and the impact of new HIV/AIDS education and whether it has resulted in any lifestyle changes by the crafts women.'[22] Wells has had to balance carefully this objective research interest with her hands-on assistance for small-scale enterprise development, because the two activities are so entwined.

When I interviewed the lead doll-maker, Lobolile Ximba, in August 2006, I asked her what was more important – the sales income or the health message

– and she replied cannily, 'It's more the message, but because that also helps to sell more dolls'. Promoting this unique selling point is far from being a cynical marketing exercise; rather it suggests a pragmatic recognition by Lobolile that the health, financial and educational prospects of her community are inter-linked, but income survival is paramount. Lobolile won the prestigious Brett Kebble Craft Award in 2004 for the best craft in South Africa, and she put the monetary award into having new housing built for her family.

The position of rural craftswomen in modern Zulu society is contradictory. While they are often the principal domestic wage earner and have status on account of their expertise, they are also vulnerable to HIV infection on account of illiteracy, gender and cultural stereotypes. Many of the women have large numbers of dependants to support, often because of the AIDS fatalities in their extended family networks.

Health literacy is crucial, beginning with mother-tongue literacy. Usually the mother makes the decision whether to refer a member of her family to a traditional healer, known as a *sangoma*, or to conventional medical care, and this decision is taken instinctively. The name of the illness is not important; the cause and the form of treatment are. In traditional healing it is believed you are ill because someone living or dead is doing something to you, so you have to call on the right ancestor for help. If you go first to a conventional doctor, the sangoma will not help later. So there are big ethical problems in trying to combine the two systems. Licensing of sangomas, currently under discussion in South Africa, may lead to approved training programmes, but these could actually disempower the traditional healers in rural areas. The sangoma is a vital practitioner and intercessor in rural Zulu culture because of the belief that illness is not just of the individual body but also of the misfortunes that may befall the community as a whole. Traditional healing embraces concepts that go much wider than the Western concept of illness and, in addition to the physical aspects of being unwell, recognises disturbances within the 'pathology' of the environment. It is a fascinating way of looking at community health, and it may be conceptually pertinent to how one might view the diseases of consumerism afflicting Western societies.

The congenial space created in Siyazama retraining workshops has empow-ered the women to articulate their health concerns outside of dominant cultural taboos and at the same time introduce design innovations in their work and promote their craft through international exhibitions and trade outlets. Wells organised the workshops to be a dynamic meeting place of different interests in support of the project:

> With the lively workshop setting, the intervention included at various times undergraduate and postgraduate design students, health workers, medical doctors, isangoma (traditional healers) and izinyanga (herbalists), people

living with AIDS, anthropologists, environmental health workers, performers, musicians and sales reps from marketing outlets all working together on a number of levels.[23]

Some of the bead dolls produced privately commemorate members of the community who have contracted AIDS and died. In the workshops, the women's craft activity, critical discussion of cultural norms and sharing of health information are literally interwoven. It has proved possible to introduce a variety of health improvement measures as an integral part of the project. For example, new mothers in the project are successfully encouraged to breastfeed their babies exclusively for the first six months from birth. Many of the bead-doll tableaux that the women create explain aspects of HIV/AIDS that are affected by cultural taboos, and so these craft works become teaching aids within the community. What impressed Wells particularly in the women's artistry was how 'the process illuminated a detailed system of visual education within the boundaries of the illiterate audience, and it became a vehicle for those that could read, decode and decipher the beaded messages',[24] and this led her to the revelation that 'through their crafts they were able to comprehend, articulate and exchange complex and sensitive concepts, thereby constructing knowledge and meaning.'[25]

Kate Wells also noted, early on in the project, how the women yearn for respect and dignity. She noticed how the women became subdued when males were present and how they would open up much more when visiting the university campus than they would in their home village. She concludes that for effective health promotion in rural areas, you need to talk to gender groups separately and then talk to them together much later. The women's stories changed depending on location and evolved through a careful building of trust. Wells' Ph.D. thesis on Siyazama developed both a feminist and anthropological stance as the project evolved, and crucial to the latter was Axel Berglund's seminal work on Zulu thought systems and beliefs.[26] Because of *hlonipha*, a strict modesty etiquette that defers to the husband's family, it is unusual to get from married Zulu women the frank views that are present in Wells' thesis.

When I visited Msinga, I was initially reticent to ask 'personal' questions of the women about AIDS, but I soon found them to be very responsive and open. They are realistic about how far they can change ingrained male attitudes but are optimistic at the prospects for improving gender relations and health awareness in their children. Lobolile told me:

> I'm respected so much now that people don't like to have any function without me there. Any craftwork that is needed, they come to me for advice. The men also receive and respect me, and call me to their discussions. I show them the beautiful artwork but I'm shy to tell them about AIDS. I don't do health promotion as such, I just show them the artwork. I don't have enough power

yet to actually teach them. There are health promotion workers in Msinga who come to talk to us, but they don't make much impression. Men only talk about AIDS behind our backs and never say anything straight to our face. It's discussed in families but not outside. It's not discussed as AIDS; the illness is always related to witchcraft. But I leave health information around [pointing to poster on wall] because some of the children can read.[27]

A younger woman, Khishwephi Sithole, explained to me:

I use the health information I get in Durban. I use protection now and I pass on the message to the children. But the doll-making is not just about AIDS; it's about finding out about our culture and knowing how we live. I don't know if it's changing men's behaviour in the bedroom. But they do listen and they want to find out more about this disease.[28]

And Tholiwe Sithole, Khishwephi's mother and the elder of the group, said to me:

We used to sit around all day doing nothing, but now we can do this and children come and ask what we're doing, so we tell them they can do it one day, so they grow up with the message in them. It's very empowering that I can teach others, and when I die other people have something to remember me by. I'm very happy about that and to think I can make a difference in the world.[29]

Siyazama has shown that design can play a significant role in communicating and transferring social, cultural and health messages in rural areas. Through their craftwork, the women have sometimes managed to overcome gender stereotypes and restrictions and stimulate open talk in their communities about HIV/AIDS and sexual practices. At the same time, the economic development of the programme has taken the women's work into an international arena. The best work produced in Siyazama, purchased from the women, is amassed in a craft collection that has toured to galleries in the UK, Canada and Scandinavia, and in 2007 the work went on show in the US at Michigan State University Museum. An exhibition, however, can only tell part of the story. It was a privilege for me to see firsthand the reality of how and where the crafts are produced and to see clear evidence of their socioeconomic impact on the women and their community.

In order to convey the detail and purpose of the crafts, I now present a transcript of a taped commentary by Kate Wells[30] as she showed me round the storeroom of Siyazama artefacts:

So many women can do this craft technique that there is huge competition between them. It's an art form that can command a lot of money for them. The geometry and symbolism in the designs are extraordinary. The repetitive use of symbols across different pieces gives them an accumulative power. Siyazama is responsible for creating its own geometric AIDS symbol. I compare this to the universal AIDS symbol used, say, on billboard posters.

These are older dolls I bought in 1996 prior to the project – this one looks quaint, but the woman who made it has gone on to win the top craft award in the country. At that time the tradition had degenerated and the African Craft Centre asked me if I could help improve this doll-making. Tourists had stopped buying them. So I supplied the makers with very good beads. I remember saying in the early days in the workshops we ran, 'What about making more of the arms', though I never suggested the breasts become more prominent. They would then go home and reflect on what they'd heard and seen in the workshops.

These are the pieces that went off to the Natural History Museum. This one is the lovemaking couple in bed. And this piece is about virginity testing by a sangoma [an annual ritual that predetermines abstinence in young Zulu women]. And this one is about rape – look at the horrified face – and this indicates it is a traditional healer who is doing the rape, and this is a gorgeous girl sangoma with the white beads, but the addition of coloured beads is a sign of something demonic going on here. This one tells a sad story of a woman's husband who is working away in Jo'burg, and every year he returns, but the Christmas this piece was made he had returned in a coffin – the prognosis for the wife is also bleak, as the man brought food and money home. This piece is about a little girl who is followed by a green snake, shown here with her parents and sangoma. Snakes bring messages from the ancestors, and their meaning depends on where you see one and what colour it is etc. The parents ask the sangoma, 'Why is the snake following our daughter?' It is a veil for the fact the girl is HIV positive.

This piece is about being called to be a sangoma, in which the training of novices is hard work. This sangoma can't get up, she's got HIV and is depleted. If she can't continue her training, death must be imminent. It's doubly bad because she can't answer the ancestors' call. If you're chosen by the ancestors, and if you then contract HIV/AIDS, it's demeaning to you and them. It brings added shame to a family.

There are stories too of wicked witches. This piece shows a witch who stole a baby. Her hair colour shows she connects with the ancestors but also with evil spirits, represented in these elongated Giacometti-like figures. Even the little bad spirits are like children that can control you. They are part of the *amadhlosi* [ancestor] spirit group.

This tableau tells a story of two children who can't find their parents. They go to the sangoma, who calls up the ancestors through a spirit guide lizard, and she tells them the parents have been kicked by a bird – a metaphor for death from AIDS. This piece was the first of the orphan tableaux. Here's a piece showing a young girl taking her granny to clinic but worried who will do it in future, as she is now HIV herself. Here's a young girl bringing fresh fruit to an old lady who's HIV. Older people with HIV are often ridiculed. Some pieces, though only a few, show conventional medical practices taking place.

They started depicting HIV-infected women on crosses in the early days. Later came the angels. Here are four angels made from white and see-through beads. We were talking at the time in a workshop about how to look after an HIV person. I told them about Oprah Winfrey and her interest in angels. I said, 'Do you think women could have wings?' 'Yes,' they said, 'in Zulu cosmology there are angels who bring messages from God', and they started measuring each other to guess the proportion of wings. Now they haven't stopped producing angels, and they put wings on many of the dolls now. They are just enjoying their imagination and taking risks creatively. They say they now have freedom to explore and enjoy. They have confidence in their ability.

We always encourage breastfeeding through our project too, exclusively for first six months before the gut change in the baby. So these craft pieces become teaching aids. We've had to overcome some stigma in breastfeeding associated with belief it can transmit HIV. Health researchers and native speakers from the university worked with us on this to encourage take-up of breastfeeding. It also, of course, improves mother and baby relations.

The *mbengis* [plates] have practical use as beer-pot covers and are particularly rich in meaning and skill, offering opportunities for weaving in the health messages that need to take place in the home. On some plates there's more use now of magical animal imagery – they are kind of scapegoats. The mathematics of the beads is very complex. I have got a huge long piece of fabric by this craft worker in my office, and she [Fokosile Ngema] has actually done loads of work for international exhibitions. Essentially it is making a connection with what is going on with HIV/AIDS in this country now to events back in 1909. If you look back to 1909 it was the Bhambatha rebellion, when there was a lot of death and mayhem going on in our country. What she is actually getting at is that what used to happen was that the Impi warriors were slain and left lying in the open fields, and in this heat bodies would bloat up and become enormously heavy, and to bury them would become problematical. What used to happen was they would slash them down the middle or drag them under the trees and get them out of the sun, as they were impossible to move around. What she is saying in the inscription, rather cleverly (and she is one of the oldest women in my project), is that people are afforded more sympathy and respect when they are dead from AIDS, and she likens that to what was going on in 1909. She can't read or write, this woman; she talks her story through to the school children, and they write it out on lined paper and then she takes it from them. There is no sort of indentation, capitals, dots and commas; it just runs continually.

Some of the prints promoting Siyazama exhibitions were done through a third-year student group, when we had a bit of a competition and four units of students came up with their response as to how it could work. What I like to do is use lino cutting technique, because that is a very strong technique that was previously used in our country to protest through art. For the US exhibition they have these images in black and white, and they have printed them off onto see-through sheets. They hang from the ceiling to the floor so you can see movement, and they can be recreated and updated. Essentially these images are trying to make everyone wear condoms so we are all sure about the risk of AIDS. Many rural people thought it was a toilet infection and that if you were Christian you would not get infected. Those were literally the first sorts of statements that came through in the project and from which we had to re-educate people.

The biggest cost to the project is in transporting the dolls to Durban – the women have to take three long taxi rides with only what they can carry, and up to three-quarters of their sales income can go on this. And there are also robbers and hijackers on the roads. The project has an entirely cash economy. Banks are not trusted; Lobolile was once defrauded by an unscrupulous bank teller who preyed on her illiteracy. There are problems in replicating or diversifying the work. In 2004 Wells reluctantly involved another rural women's group in Siyazama, but it did not work out. There was a lot of tension, and the new group were not skilled enough and found the quality threshold of the work too demanding. There are a growing number of retailers' requests for animal figures, but should the Siyazama women focus on the dolls alone? Will the project lose its health focus through diversity? On the other hand, making animals could retain and enrich the health storytelling element, as Zulu culture is centred on cattle and mythical animals.

The project's ongoing connection with the Durban University of Technology suggests there is much creativity to be had in research itself in devising means of evaluation that are sensitive to context while remaining academically rigorous. The university has given priority to the practical medium-term aim of developing a business plan with the women, so Wells can then stand down to a consultant role only. The women will become shareholders, and a fundraiser will be engaged. It is recognised that the project cannot survive long-term on donor funds and must become entirely income-generating for its sustainability. The project needs to become an 'incubator' in its next phase, and much more postgraduate research could be done on it then. This process has begun with a one-year partnership of Siyazama and Durban University of Technology with the Department of Industrial Arts and Design at Makerere University in Uganda and the School of Design of Northumbria University in North East England. The initiative explored the marketability of health-themed craft artefacts, and it was funded by the England–Africa Partnership of the UK government's Department for Innovation, Universities and Skills.[31]

Siyazama's success is due in no small way to how 'big city ideas' on health and enterprise have been introduced sensitively into a traditional rural context, with the women's welfare guarded by a consistent ethics of practice. Both skills development and health education seem to have never been forced, and the women have been allowed to pass on their learning in their own way, at their own pace.


## THE CURRICULUM DEVELOPMENT PROJECT, JOHANNESBURG

I also wanted to see, by contrast, how arts in health might be undertaken in a challenging urban context, where education might be a more formal require- ment for delivery of the work. So on both my visits to South Africa in preparation for this book, I spent time with the Curriculum Development Project (CDP). CDP is a non-government arts in education agency based in the rundown (but soon to be regenerated) district of Bertrams in Johannesburg, where the soccer World Cup takes place in 2010. CDP's founder members were artists and activists who, from the 1970s onwards, taught children in back yards, garages and church halls. Under the aegis of 'black consciousness', many youths were beginning to discover that although they had been dispossessed, they had a voice, and it could be used. As CDP's director, Charlotte Schaer, explained to me, that voice found expression mainly in theatre workshops and poetry groups in the townships, combining acting, words, music and dance, using styles and techniques taken from township life. This expression reached a critical state with the eruption of Soweto in June 1976, which was the result of a long-standing dissatisfaction with children having to learn in the Afrikaans language of the oppressor.

The community arts movement reflected, and even helped develop, the resistance that was taking over the streets by June 1976. Expression found new outlets in graphics and on T-shirts and posters. Community-based arts projects included a strong focus on teaching art, and often classes centred on encourag- ing young adults to find a political and social voice. Either the absolute lack of arts education in the schools or a culturally biased curriculum led to teachers wanting to give some creative outlet to children. This rebellious arts education aimed to break down the more rigidly defined Western distinctions between discrete disciplines and offer insights into the roots of discrimination.

In 1986, four years before the CDP was legally constituted, a few art teachers implemented a project in Soweto at a time when the township's population was barricaded in by the army. It was called the Khula Udweba, a Zulu phrase meaning 'draw as you grow and grow as you draw'. These teachers developed new curricula and trained young artists and schoolteachers who had never before had access to teaching art. Graduates from this course joined the CDP

Trust in 1992. Since then the CDP members have delivered arts and culture education and training to hundreds of teachers and artists, benefiting thousands of children from preschool to informal structures.[32] The main underpinning principles of the CDP training curriculum remain to:

➤ promote an understanding and appreciation of the value of arts and culture in social development, in reclaiming and making identity, in community health and healing, in addressing harmful stereotyping and racist practice and in skills development

➤ train teachers who have had little or no art training or experience in various creative teaching and practical art making methods,

➤ implement a participative learner-centred teaching practice to counteract the rigid authoritarian modes of the past

➤ bring the creative experience of the arts to as many learners as possible

➤ encourage and promote South African and African arts and culture practices within a global context.

CDP's work, and that of many other non-government organisations (NGOs), remains rooted in those early civil society responses to a harsh political climate, affirming the arts as vehicles for social transformation, for addressing crucial community health issues (especially the HIV/AIDS epidemic), for presenting alternatives to violence and its impact on children, for building social cohesion and, of course, for providing every child with the opportunity to achieve his or her fullest creative potential.

Charlotte Schaer feels that delivery on CDP's principles is increasingly hampered by ideological as well as fiscal constraints. In her view, as presented in a paper to an education conference at Durham University in 2008,[33] the South African Department of Education has made a critical error in focusing on curriculum content and change within a UK-influenced outcomes-based model while neglecting the fact that the vast majority of teachers have totally inadequate training in the arts. Arts education consequently remains low on the government's list of priorities.

With dwindling mainstream support, CDP struggles to provide a structured course for around 50 teachers a year, accredited through the University of the Witwatersrand, disseminating arts in education techniques that try to produce work of quality with the bare minimum of resources. Schaer passionately believes that interventions by NGOs, even though ever diminishing, are critical to communal well-being, and that participation in the arts promotes sharing and caring, and informed and economically viable communities and schools.

Where Schaer feels CDP can take heart is that the arts in all their forms seem to be more prevalent in community development and informal training contexts than ever before. The impetus amongst the NGO sector to view the arts as a vital instrument in social change has not waned, and its very resilience testifies to the validity of community arts practice in both a national and international context. CDP has in recent years mobilised itself to address the plight of economic migrants and trauma victims from Zimbabwe, who live precariously in CDP's local district – just some of the three million refugees from Mugabe's regime thought to be living in South Africa. In May 2008, resentment of the immigrants turned to outright violence, forcing thousands of Zimbabweans in Johannesburg and the townships to seek refuge in police stations and churches.[34]

## FROM BERTRAMS TO BEADWORK

My trips to South Africa set out ideas for future collaboration between CAHHM at Durham University and some of the organisations I visited. In 2007 my colleague Mary Robson, artist and NESTA fellow, led a team to Bertrams in Johannesburg to undertake a short residency with CDP in order to help develop a skills resource with invited participants – schoolteachers, preschool practitioners and librarians. It proved to be a valuable mutual learning experience, as well as relevant to the training needs of the participants. The residency was designed as an informal, exploratory project to compare and share approaches to achieving meaningful practice in arts in health and education, and it was also intended to be the basis for further exchanges.

Mary was accompanied by Dawn Williams, coordinator of the Creative Partnerships national co-mentoring programme for teachers and artists known as Reflect, and by two specialist early-years teachers in creative arts from King Edward's School in North Shields. Early-years education in South Africa is very different from the UK model. There are some state preschools, but they are in the minority compared with the thousands of informal or individually owned preschools.

Mary kept a weblog[35] of the visit as the basis for an assessment report on the residency to assist CAHHM's ongoing research into the health benefits of arts education projects that aim to develop emotional literacy.

Nineteen women turned up for the workshop. Some were teachers, some ran their own crèches, and a couple of them were local artists. The workshop began with introductions, and in pairs and then fours conversations developed. There was much laughter as participants swapped lone words of Zulu, Afrikaans and Geordie, and by the time they got to the preliminary exercise of drawing with their eyes closed, hysteria was in the air. Shrieks of laughter set the tone for the week. As Mary commented:

> The atmosphere made for the beginnings of deeper conversations. Relationships were being nurtured. We seemed to move a huge emotional distance in a few hours. We could talk as we worked next to each other. Someone started singing *Frere Jacques* and then the challenge was on. French, English, Afrikaans and

Zulu versions ensued. And then, a heart-stopping moment; Nancy was sitting with her chin in her hand and began to sing *Nkosi Sikele Africa*. Without a pause and whilst still working, the whole room joined in. Then songs were tumbling out from all sides of the room. Songs we had in common, some we'd never heard but seemed familiar. There is something about this singing. It is, in the moment, pure community. Some sing along, some harmonise. Some, like us, hum along as best they know. It is magnetic, pulling everyone into a space that can be intensely emotional and yet boundaried by the song itself. Nancy must have had a reason, a thought, a notion to sing that song then. It most certainly wasn't to impress us. It wasn't performance. It is part of the fabric of life. For Dawn and I, this echoed our long-held belief that congenial space is a vital characteristic of the way we work.[36]

The early-years teachers had brought with them from the UK some story sacks they had designed, containing props to illustrate fables, rhymes and numeracy games. The task was then for three groups to each make a storytelling sack that would be left at the CDP centre and to take away the makings of one for themselves. The participants were passionate and so committed to the cause of helping young preschool children that nothing was too much effort. There was not a shred of cynicism. Everything offered was grasped and learned from and within hours applied back at their schools.

Although the weeklong residency had an arts in education focus, an under-lying purpose was to assess the potential of developing health-themed work in a primary-school context. That potential seemed enormous, as evidenced by a visit later to Nancy Kubu's school, the wonderfully named Land of Joy in Soweto. Mary described the visit thus:

We arrived at a set of low, brick buildings surrounding a courtyard with a covered walkway. The walkway held three hundred children aged between 1 and 6, the whole school, and their teachers. The minute we got out of the car, they erupted in joyous song. We stood there, glued to the spot, and drank it in.

*Land of Joy in Soweto,*
*Come and join us today*
*This is colour yellow!*
*This is colour red!*
*Colour blue!*
*Colour green!*
*Come and join us today!*
*Keep up the good work and shine!*

After they dispersed, Nancy took us on a tour of the classes. Sixty or so happy, confident, nurtured children to a room and not a chair or a table in sight.

Heather commented: 'I will never complain again about the lack of resources in my classroom'. Every room was drenched in song. The little ones, standing amongst their cots, danced and sang a bumblebee song. Older children marched and balanced to *This is the Way to London Town*. The eldest children recited 'Do you know that children have rights and needs?' and then proceeded to list their declaration. We met the cook and her assistant cooking fish and rice for lunch. Small flower beds with irises and succulents were being carefully tended by a gardener. Everywhere you looked, something was being nurtured. And on Nancy's office wall, on a sheet of paper protected by polythene, the following list:

*This year I will grow*
*This year I will focus*
*This year I will surprise myself*
*This year I will build*
*This year I will try something new*
*This year I will be free*
*This year I will make changes*
*This year I will dare and do*

Over tea, Nancy showed us photographs of the school's progress from being based in her home to the present buildings, pointing out the teachers who have passed away and the elders who take care of their parentless grandchildren. She arranges trips for the elders to recognise their contribution to the community. The school is open from 6.00am until 5.00pm with transport provided to get the children there. If there are any children left at the end of the day, she takes them to her home until they are collected. We left The Land Of Joy with children's farewells ringing in our ears.[37]

Mary then moved on to Durban to meet Dr Kate Wells and the Siyazama doll-makers. The craftswomen were coming in to the university for a day of conversation, making and marketplace activities and to meet Mary. They came from two different parts of the KwaZulu-Natal province, from Msinga and The Valley of A Thousand Hills. The women arrived with their mats and towels, ignored the chairs and set up camp on the floor of the staffroom. They got out their current work and began beading. Mary commented in her weblog that:

I was asking questions of them as individuals but soon realised that they thought in a much more communal way. They are not a collective as such but one will represent another, take dolls and deliver her wages, irrespective of the amount. Kate and her colleagues met with each of the women in turn, doing the business of the market place. Their mutual regard was apparent; an ease developed over the years in spite of a lack of mutual language.[38]

Mary also kept a record of her conversations with Charlotte Schaer and colleagues at CDP. Schaer explained that the suppression of culture had been a strategy of the apartheid regime. Because culture was closely allied to the arts and its power was recognised, access to arts education was denied for all communities except whites. In 1996, however, when the education system was being redefined, those newly in power were adamant that arts and culture be separated because, in Schaer's words, 'culture is political, the arts can be technical'. But she felt that in the field of arts and community health, arts and culture cannot be separated, and trying to separate them would be an energy-sapping and fruitless task because they are intertwined in a most complicated way.

To establish common ground with one another, Charlotte Schaer and Mary set out the characteristics of their practice and principles. These were remarkably attuned and similar to those I described in Chapter 3. They agreed the following as the basis of their work in arts in community health:

➤ that reflective processes are inherent and bring with them responsibilities for what you might do, your role in it and your place in other people's lives
➤ that we come into a project or activity with privilege so we cannot be in the participants' shoes as we have not experienced their experience
➤ that we are responsive; that we do everything possible not to misrepresent the authentic voices of the voiceless, and are careful not to presume that vulnerable people are completely voiceless
➤ we don't go out to dispense; we go out to give
➤ our work is necessarily and proudly interventionist but mindful of history, dignity and boundaries
➤ our work requires a safe and stimulating environment, a congenial space, because an inappropriate environment can result in people feeling they have nothing to give, yet anything that anyone brings is pertinent
➤ the very act of creating something can be transformative because 'art is political, healing and subversive, and the making of it takes you to subconscious, spiritual places where it is a very deep meditation' (Schaer)
➤ 'finding the way through' is a constant mantra because 'a lot of pressure comes from sheer survival and the struggle to keep this work alive is related to its intensity so we have very high standards' (Schaer)
➤ to be organic, flexible and responsive is not random; the work is structured and rigorous
➤ we practise unconditional positive regard and are appropriately non-judgmental in order to facilitate empathy
➤ the importance of relationship, of person-centred practice, means we are attentive to the spaces between people, the subtle exchanges of energy that can occur, sometimes non-verbal.[39]

## FUTURE COLLABORATIONS

Several elements were identified that could shape future collaborations with CDP and the Siyazama project. Ever since I first visited CDP and showed pictures of our community lantern events, Charlotte Schaer had been determined to somehow produce an inner-city Johannesburg equivalent and to explore, in particular, how to involve the refugee community at a time of tension. Kate Wells visited a lanterns event on Tyneside in 2003 and had expressed a similar wish to include lanterns in the Siyazama project.

The story sacks produced in the residency at CDP were inspirational to practitioners and suggested that the experience could be built on. King Edward's School and Creative Partnerships (Tyneside) were keen to be involved in any future dissemination and collaboration that might develop from this visit. Through CAHHM, we began to arrange learning events at the Wolfson Research Institute from 2008 that bring together the Tyneside schools in the Creative Partnerships initiative that we have been working with, as well as other schools-based arts and health projects in North East England and Yorkshire that are described in the next case example.

Thanks to a one-off donation from a Durham University alumnus, we were able to invite Charlotte Schaer and two of her colleagues in CDP, along with Nancy from The Land Of Joy, to the UK in spring 2008. Their visit included taking part in the annual Lanternland workshops and celebration at Chickenley School in Dewsbury, where Mary has been resident artist since 2003. This was so they could gain understanding of the techniques of lantern-making and event management and could begin to think of how it might work back in Johannesburg. Schaer was asked to speak at the first of our Wolfson Institute events, and her colleagues were also invited to King Edward's School to establish a firm twinning link. A few weeks later Kate Wells came to Tyneside to open a Siyazama exhibition at the University of Northumbria. We both spoke at an international colloquium there on the subject of design and health, and we made plans for a future joint project.

In August 2008, Mary revisited CDP in Johannesburg to instigate a small-scale lanterns event in the Bertrams district, drawing participants from the local community, from invited voluntary groups and schools and from a refugee theatre group from Harare. This event was intended as a precursor to a much bigger one to take place in 2009, providing an opportunity to experiment with local materials to produce lanterns that might have a distinct African feel. Mary then went on to Durban University of Technology to work with Kate Wells' graphic design students in developing from paper-cuts some design ideas for prototype large-scale doll lanterns. The aim is to fuse UK craft techniques with South African ones, using wire, rattan, willow and fabric to create semi-permanent structures that can be electrically lit. The resultant artworks are to be used as an impetus for further creative work by the students and exhibited as powerful symbols of the Siyazama project.

From these initial exchanges of thought and practice around arts, education and community health, there is now a cross-cultural collaboration moving along what I call 'the lantern road', which is the subject of the next chapter of case examples.

## REFERENCES

1 Marmot M. *Status Syndrome: how your social standing directly affects your health and life expectancy*. London: Bloomsbury; 2004.

2 Putnam R. *Bowling Alone: the collapse and revival of American community*. New York: Simon and Schuster; 2000.

3 Dodgy Clutch Theatre. *Elephant: a simple tale*. Newcastle: Dodgy Clutch; 2008.

4 Mandela N. *Long Walk to Freedom*. London: Abacus; 1995.

5 Johnson RW. *South Africa: the first man, the last nation*. London: Weidenfield and Nicholson; 2004.

6 Mbeki T. Fourth Annual Nelson Mandela Lecture [speech]. 29 July 2006. Available at: www.anc.org.za/ancdocs/history/mbeki/2006/index.html (accessed 5 August 2008).

7 Kaiser Family Foundation. *South Africa*. Available at: www.globalhealthreporting.org/countries/countrypage.asp?collID=11&id=37 (accessed 5 August 2008).

8 Barnett T, Whiteside A. *AIDS in the Twenty-First Century: disease and globalisation*. London: Palgrave Macmillan; 2002. p. 11.

9 Health Systems Trust. Available at: www.hst.org.za/publications/437 (accessed 5 January 2009).

10 UNAIDS. *New Data on Male Circumcision and HIV Prevention*: policy and programming implications. Montreux: UNAIDS; 2007.

11 Nattrass N. *The Moral Economy of AIDS in South Africa*. Cambridge: Cambridge University Press; 2004.

12 Whiteside A, Sunter C. *AIDS: the challenge for South Africa*. Cape Town: Human and Rousseau Tafelberg; 2000.

13 www.soulcity.org.za (accessed 19 May 2005).

14 Kelly K, Parker W, Hajiyiannis H, *et al. Tsha Tsha: key findings of the evaluation*. Johannesburg: Centre for AIDS Development Research and Evaluation; 2005.

15 UNAIDS. *UNAIDS Communication Framework on HIV/AIDS: a new direction*. New York: UNAIDS/Penn State University; 1999.

16 White M. Establishing common ground in community-based arts in health. *J R Soc Promot Health*. 2006; **126**(3): 128–33.

17 www.dramaide.co.za/contentpage.aspx?pageid=2194 (accessed 27 July 2005).

18 Dalrymple L. DramAidE: An Evaluation of Interactive Drama and Theatre for HIV/AIDS Education in South Africa. *Proceedings of the Exeter International Conference: Drama as Social Intervention*; 2005 April; University of Exeter. p. 11.

19 Sachs A. Preparing ourselves for freedom: culture and the ANC constitutional guidelines. *TDR*. 1991; **35**(1): 187–93.

20 Medilinks. *Talking about HIV/AIDS: the loveLife campaign*. 12 October 2001. Available at: www.medilinkz.org/news/news2.asp?NewsID=232 (accessed 5 August 2008).

21 Tech Express. *Siyazama*. Durban: Durban University of Technology; 2001.

22 Wells K. *Manipulating Metaphors: an analysis of beadwork crafts as a contemporary medium for communicating on AIDS and culture in KwaZulu-Natal*. Durban: Durban University of Technology; 2006. p. 24.

23 Ibid. p. 30.

24 Ibid. p. 31.

25 Ibid. p. 37.

26 Berglund A. *Zulu Thought Patterns and Symbolism*. Indiana: Indiana University Press: 1989.

27 Ximba L. Taped interview. 12 August 2006.

28 Sithole K. Taped interview. 12 August 2006.

29 Sithole T. Taped interview. 12 August 2006.

30 Wells K. Taped interview. 2 September 2005.

31 England–Africa Partnership. *Design, Health and Community*. Newcastle: University of Northumbria; 2008.

32 Solomon LA. *Creative Beginnings: a hands-on innovative approach to art making for adults and children*. Johannesburg: Curriculum Development Project; 2005.

33 Schaer C. *An Historical Context of the Struggle for Arts in Education in South Africa before and after Apartheid, with Reference to the Roles of Non Governmental Organisations*. Durham: University of Durham (CAHHM); 2008.

34 Thousands seek sanctuary as South Africans turn on refugees. *Guardian*. 20 May 2008.

35 Robson M. Social Pedagogy in the Rainbow Nation. Weblog available at: http://mjrobson.typepad.com/mary_robson/.

36 Ibid.

37 Ibid.

38 Ibid.

39 Ibid.

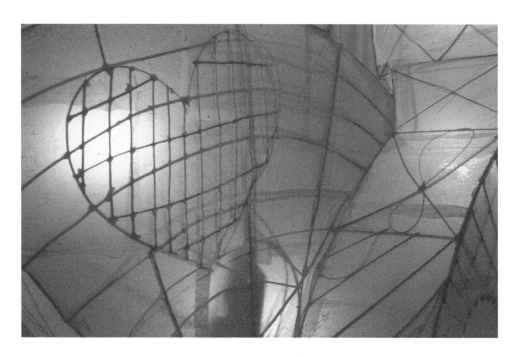

Lantern detail. PHOTO: CENTRE FOR ARTS AND HUMANITIES IN HEALTH AND MEDICINE

# CHAPTER 7

# The lantern road: case examples from Northern England

Candles burning
Children laughing
Rain dropping
Lanterns flopping
Wind howling
Dogs growling
For the lights of hearts
. . . were glowing.

The Wrekenton lanterns rap

Lantern parades have been a connecting thread of imagery throughout my 20 years' involvement in arts in health projects. They have provided milestones that myself and some close colleagues have used to chart the development and direction of the kind of transformational social projects that cultural critic Raymond Williams defined as producing 'resources for a journey of hope'.[1] They are, literally, occasions to view a community in another light. Sometimes they are one-off events, but in many cases they have become annual celebrations and part of wider programmes of work that connect arts, health education and community development.

Some of the projects I review in these case examples from northern England, such as Roots and Wings and Looking Well Healthy Living Centre, provide small-scale but significant practical instances of how social capital is produced and built upon. Lantern events can provide a tangible picture of how that capital is in circulation in the community. They create potent, resonating images for times and places, and they throw light upon what makes for healthy living. Every neighbourhood should have one.

The use of handmade lanterns in the UK for celebratory processions origi-nated with Welfare State International (WSI), with whom I worked in the 1980s. In August 1982 the company performed at an international theatre festival in Toga-mura, Japan. While there, director John Fox and other company members came by chance upon a spectacular and inspirational carnival parade know as the Sea Lanterns Procession, consisting of large illuminated floats carried by villagers. The bearers descended woodland slopes to the sea and launched the floats with joyous ceremony.[2] WSI had for years used handmade lanterns to delineate outdoor ballroom space for barn dancing, but seeing in Japan how they could be used for a whole community performance presented as a 'living' artwork was a revelation.

Meanwhile back in Cumbria, WSI artist Alison Jones was coincidentally experimenting with creating lanterns from willow and paper that could be carried by whole communities. She and fellow artist Gill Bond then devised a lantern design that was tried out for the first time in the company's visual theatre work *Scarecrow Zoo* which was presented in November 1982 at Bracknell South Hill Park Arts Centre. This use of processional lights combined with the traditional Japanese festival provided an inspirational confluence of ideas for developing a seminal community arts event.

In September 1983 the first annual lantern procession took place in WSI's home town of Ulverston in Cumbria as part of the newly created Charter Week celebrations that reaffirmed Ulverston's status as a market town. Alison Jones, with the assistance of Mo Cumbo, prepared the first procession as a small-scale event, as most of the company were away working on a spectacle for the London International Festival of Theatre. This event introduced community participants to the simple pyramid lantern, carried on a small bamboo cane, which has since become the staple image in lantern processions.

The procession then grew in scale each year, and by the late 1980s tour-ism brochures were referring to the 'traditional lantern-making' of Ulverston. The event continues to this day, and it has inspired many similar proces-sions elsewhere, working to different themes and contexts. For example, the now-legendary lanterns of the annual Slaithwaite Moonraking Festival in West Yorkshire were developed by WSI artists Gill Bond and Andy Burton soon after the first Ulverston parade. And in 2003 ex-WSI artists in Walk the Plank arts company orchestrated a finale spectacle of hundreds of lanterns around a giant illuminated figure as a conclusion to the Commonwealth Games in Manchester.

As repeated events in a social calendar, lantern processions have established particularly strong roots with communities in the north of England. In 1987 Alison Jones reported that:

> People have described the [Ulverston] lantern procession as a 'river of light' so

I have decided to go with this analogy concentrating mainly on the notion of 'reflections' – the lantern as a reflection of oneself, whatever that may be, literal or abstract. This is most successful; it is understood and interpreted in many ways and exquisite lanterns have resulted.[3]

As community involvement in the Ulverston lanterns doubled in size by the second year, artists Liz Lynch and Mary Robson were recruited to assist. They quickly noted that the event was much more than a participatory visual theatre piece by WSI:

> The procession is the event. It has always been about a process that begins when someone sees the poster, hears the word, and comes to a workshop. That process is complex (involving things social and aesthetic as well as practical) and joyous. The product is the procession; carrying a lantern that you have made through your streets, in front of your friends. The product is by, with and for the procession and its participants. It is now apparent that the ending should reflect the ultimately personal nature of the event.[4]

These observations were at the root of both Alison's and Mary's subsequent interest in adapting lantern events to health promotion contexts. They realised that lanterns permitted a discreet externalisation of personal feelings within a neighbourhood spectacle, building social cohesion and identity and releasing inner tensions. The open conversations that occurred about health issues in the workshops, the intergenerational working, the personal meanings invested in lanterns and the beneficial activities intrinsic to the event of a brisk walk and homemade soup and bread all provided a microcosm of healthy living. In 1988 I invited West Midlands GP Dr Malcolm Rigler to the Ulverston procession, and with Alison Jones' help, he subsequently developed a similar event at his Withymoor practice.

I had noted in the previous year the effect the lantern parade was having on the Ulverston community in generating an image of its integration and adaptation, as follows:

> On lantern night, hundreds of families assemble at dusk with their lanterns, or rather illuminated images drawn from the local ecology: marine life, flowers, mythical sea beasts, waves, clouds and mountains, clock towers and lighthouses, the pole star, and even submarines. The parade begins with several small processions around local neighbourhoods, stopping off at elderly people's sheltered housing to collect their lanterns to be borne by children. Each procession slowly threads its way to the town centre, where they all merge and weave into a river of light bobbing above the heads of the participants, to the accompaniment of carnival percussion orchestras and the town brass band.

Virtually everyone turns out for the event. En masse, these simple lanterns are an extraordinary, animated artwork that would be impossible to exhibit in a gallery or price as a commodity. They exist only for a few hours through a great deal of collective involvement and imagination. The event transmits its visual poetry across generations and enables the community to affirm itself in a spirit of fun and hope before the coming of each winter.[5]

This was for me the beginning of 'the lantern road', a recurrent image of arts in community health that has imprinted itself on my retinas for over 20 years. In this chapter, I want to retrace my steps through some of the locations where that road has led.

## WREKENTON 'HAPPY HEARTS'

As I explained in Chapter 1, this event began as the culmination of a two-year intergenerational arts in health programme. The Happy Hearts celebratory lantern parade for the Wrekenton and Springwell estates in Gateshead became an annual event that took place each March from 1994 to 2006. Alison Jones and Mary Robson were the lead artists on the first year's event. When it became clear there was local interest to make it an annual 'tradition', the management of the event passed to Mary, working with local sculptor Gilly Rogers. Core support came from Gateshead Libraries and Arts Service, with a succession of charitable trusts and sponsors providing one-off grants. In time, the estates' residents also helped to fundraise for the procession under the organisational umbrella of Happy Hearts Alliance.

From the outset the event involved hundreds of local children and their families, voluntary agencies, churches and the district health promotion team. Wrekenton is an area that is unfairly regarded as a 'black spot' in terms of both its health profile and the media's image of it as a rough place. In my experience of working there, however, it is a caring and imaginative community with resilient good humour. Over the years the procession became the distinctive event in the local calendar, a metaphorical 'screening' and celebration of community health.

A healthy heart theme originated out of a public health report on Gateshead in 1992 that identified the borough as having the worst morbidity rate in coronary heart disease in England.[6] Other health problems in the community that were evident to the artists working on the lantern project included a high use of antibiotics, problems with diet and obesity. The number of visits to the doctor was very high among women in Wrekenton, and the ward also had a high rate of teenage pregnancy.

The base for the project was Wrekenton's Fell Dyke primary school, selected by the artists on account of the local knowledge and dynamic energy of the staff and also because of the school's community room, which enabled the event to engage families as well as the schoolchildren. Mary Robson grasped the potential of this from the outset:

> The lantern workshops became a congenial space. Slowly, a gang of women and the occasional man became involved. The power of chat became the conduit for discussion of health, life and death that was sometimes serious, at others hysterical. At the centre of it all was the art and activity of lantern making. Parents would come to help their child make one and would still be coming days after that one had been finished. From simple materials came magical objects.[7]

Importantly, it was not just the schoolchildren and their immediate families who were involved. Teachers, health professionals and local artists learned how to make lanterns at an open day held for all interested parties. The project team attended Wrekenton network meetings – schools, churches, community education, social services, the youth service, libraries, health visitors and the police were all represented. From these meetings came more support for the project, with the involvement of the neighbouring St Oswald's Catholic Primary School. The local community education project would produce the poster, and the community policeman would organise the route and arrange security and traffic management for the parade.

As well as lanterns, the Wrekenton event included making fruit pictures with nursery children (to introduce them to a variety of fresh fruits), making of wholemeal bread baked in an outdoor sculptural kiln by a local baker, and lantern songs and raps composed by the children. In the two-week preparation period of lantern-making, health information would be imparted and shared in a relaxed and domestic manner:

> The common denominator between school, lantern workshop and Health Promotion Bus is that each can induce wariness. To voluntarily step over the threshold into unfamiliar territory can seem a daunting challenge – especially when there is a possibility of confirming an image of poor health and education. By holding the lantern workshops in the community rooms of a school, and by including the Health Promotion personnel in the team, we made the whole experience informal and less of a threat.[8]

Lanterns are made from willow sticks and wet-strength tissue paper coated with latex and lit by candles. As dusk falls, they are revealed as having delicate, lacy structures. Glowing amber, they bob along on an incoming tide of darkness, each having its place in the collective stream; none is dispensable. The centrepiece of the Wrekenton procession each year was the giant 'heart of community' lantern, which at the end of the event was placed on a hill and illuminated with pyrotechnics, looking like a large belated valentine. The resonance of this finale image was widely commented on by local people at the end of each year's event. As a local teacher's husband, who had a heart condition, once observed to me, 'seeing that big heart light up made my heart feel better', and a nine-year-old boy subsequently wrote, 'When the lanterns light up, everyone turns into my friend.'[9]

That sense of metaphor is important. The core of this event, and a typical characteristic of arts in community health work, is the nurturing of emotional intelligence and informal learning. The association of good times and positive self-image with an ephemeral arts event and its processes is a potent one. As the deputy head of Fell Dyke School said to Mary Robson after the first year's event, 'When you came here and said "We're all going to make lanterns out of sticks and glue and walk down the streets with them", well, I thought you were mad. I'd never have believed what I've seen tonight. Look, it's Friday night in Wrekenton and everybody's eating brown bread and soup, and enjoying it!'[10] Aside from the hearty occasion, the enduring impact is in the after-image – the one of the big heart on the hill – that is left in the mind's eye. This is a rite of transformation, not just for the people involved but for the streets as well. Participants gained confidence for themselves and for where they came from. The event's workshops provided a space from which latent talents could emerge.

Over the years, developments occurred that could not have been planned for. Each lantern had the image of a heart secreted into it by its maker. Special lanterns were made for newborn babies and for those residents who had recently died. In 1996 a beautiful pony lantern was gifted, by invitation, to Dunblane Library as a symbol of solidarity, as Dunblane's community had been traumatised by the shooting of children in their local primary school. And on a more mundane level, lantern-making had an important social role in enabling people to call a truce on local quarrels; as one Wrekenton woman pointed out, 'Some of us don't get on. But at Lanterns we put all that to one side. You see each other different at Lanterns'.[11]

For a long time, the relationships forged around the arts activity ensured the undiminished energy of the Wrekenton neighbourhood to develop and reinforce its healthy living message each year. It was never easy, however, as each year posed new challenges for the funding and infrastructure of the event. The already dilapidated condition of the school's workshop rooms was aggravated further by repeated ram-raids and arson attacks. That part of the school was closed down, and for a few years the workshop base had a nomadic existence, moving from one community hall to another, each proving problematic. In the Community Centre, for example, lantern-making had to share the workshop room with computer training, and the local Methodist hall was an ideal space but would not permit the complementary therapy of shiatsu massage, which had become a staple of the event for both mothers and children.

In 2002 the rebuilt primary school opened new community rooms, funded through the government's one-off Space for Sports and Arts fund. In 2003, the tenth anniversary of the event, a film of both workshops and procession was made with support from Arts Council England, involving young people in its production.[12] Also in that year, a qualitative research study supported by the King's Fund and the Nuffield Trust, published by CAHHM, examined Happy Hearts in detail.[13]

By 2004 the event was sufficiently well established for it to be the lead project in a proposed longitudinal study into arts in community health. This was to be developed by CAHHM through the creation of a cluster programme with other similar projects that the Happy Hearts team of artists had instigated elsewhere in the region.[14] Long-term, closely focused development work appeared to be the key to success, revealing the lanterns event to be rich in both local mythology and objective data for undertaking participatory evaluation of the health gain and cost benefits.

Local volunteers were receiving training in managing arts in health events and had become advocates of the work to other communities. A peer-group training programme was underway with Wrekenton residents, assisting communities on estates in nearby Sunderland and the west end of Newcastle who wanted to develop 'health lanterns' and link up with each other. After a few rocky years, the project seemed to have found renewed vigour and vision, but then it faltered again.

From humble beginnings, Happy Hearts had become a nationally renowned project and an example of good arts in health practice. It was featured in conference presentations around the world and at a seminar on social inclusion held in Downing Street. It had quickly progressed from a single event into a robust annual tradition. Local people took it to their hearts, commemorating important occasions in their lives through it and becoming expert lantern-makers in the process.

When Happy Hearts began, there was a wealth of networking activity in Wrekenton, but in the last two years of the event the picture became quite different. Fundraising had proved more and more difficult, but the biggest concern was the sudden falling-off of community contacts and meaningful development. It became a battle to get the event to happen at all. There were lots of reasons for this: broad community network meetings no longer happened; changes of staff in the schools and local voluntary agencies, as well as externally imposed changes in their outcome targets, produced less of an emphasis on the social development aspects of the project; the police began charging a considerable fee to come on the parade; and while people from other communities were coming to observe and be involved in the project, it was evident that fewer new local people were signing up to its potential. The aim of Happy Hearts had been to work within a community network to help promote inner strength, health and development on every level. It was essentially about sharing. It could only happen in the context of a constantly developing tapestry of relationships, and when it was no longer supported by a strong local network it could not continue. The organisers felt it would be a contradiction in terms for it to do so, and they regretfully closed down the event in 2006.

By the 1990s, lantern procession instigators Mary Robson and Alison Jones had learned that arts in community health needed a stronger infrastructure than just participation and goodwill. It is interesting to see how some other lantern parades fared. These were inspired partly by Wrekenton's example and partly by Mary and Alison's search for fertile contexts in which to explore both practice and research into what emotionally binds communities together.

## SUNDERLAND 'CATCH THE LIGHT'

Shortly before the demise of lanterns at Wrekenton, the perfect school for the continuation of such an event had been found. Southwick Primary School in Sunderland is in the midst of an area that has undergone radical regeneration since the millennium. Over five years, a large proportion of the local housing stock was demolished, displacing hundreds of people and splitting up extended families who had lived near to each other for generations. School rolls fell as a result, with one primary school closing and the remaining pupils transferring to continue their education at Southwick.

In 2000, Common Knowledge, CAHHM's arts in health learning programme for Tyne and Wear Health Action Zone, developed a relationship with Southwick Primary through a residency by visual artist Chris Hollis. This residency aimed to assist with the development of a 'friendship garden' and the provision of exterior and interior murals. At the same time, Mary Robson led training sessions with staff on the development of emotional literacy. Southwick staff and parents then visited the Wrekenton Happy Hearts lanterns event in 2002. Wrekenton women made them a 'friendship lantern' in the workshop, and it is carried to this day on the Sunderland procession. Friendships were begun with Wrekenton residents as some Southwick volunteers helped with stewarding and got a good idea of the organisation and issues involved in a night-time event. They could easily see how the idea could be adapted for their own community.

The head teacher and staff of Southwick Primary recognised that self-esteem in their community – both individual and communal – was very low. There was a perceived need to re-energise the community. They believed a lanterns event would symbolise the bringing of light and hope to their area. It would commemorate the old housing and community and celebrate the new one rising from the demolition site. It was to demonstrate, as head teacher Trish Stoker put it, 'that underneath, the heart of the community is still beating. It will show that we still care.' The recurring imagery in this event is that of stars and houses, and this forms a finale tableau that is illuminated in the schoolyard at the conclusion of the procession. Most of all, the event celebrates Southwick Primary's year-round work on emotional literacy, reinforcing its commitment to the Healthy Schools Standard.

The first Southwick lantern procession took place in October 2003. Funding was raised from a variety of sources, including trusts, regeneration initiatives and the local authority. The first event involved some 150 children and their families from both schools, and it has grown since then to encompass the wider community living in the new housing stock. The artists from Happy Hearts run training sessions for staff and parents, and all work together in the workshops. Chris Hollis has regularly returned to work with pupils and parents to create a unique record of the event in photographs and sketches that led to other permanent artworks, including a commissioned oil painting by Chris of the first procession.

Southwick Primary is part of the Creative Partnerships arts in education initiative for Sunderland and North Durham, and this extra resource has ensured that the lanterns experience exerts influence on arts practice throughout the school year. The head and governors are fully committed to continuing Catch The Light and wish it to become, literally, the school's beacon on its new site.

## LOOKING WELL

Alison Jones grasped early on that arts in community health needed a 'home' from which to radiate and from which to draw in new energy. She consequently spent the late 1990s establishing Looking Well, an arts-led healthy living centre in her home town of Bentham, North Yorkshire. Her own practice developed from her training as a theatre designer but later extended to working in health through community arts and celebratory event-making. As her groundbreaking pilot projects in primary healthcare settings became a full-time occupation, she formed a business partnership in 1990 with poster artist John Angus producing health promotion materials to commission. At the same time she continued to work in socially deprived areas in the West Midlands and the North East, where she pioneered the role and value of the arts in promoting the health of individuals and communities.

By the mid-1990s she was disillusioned, facing increasing demand for her services nationwide but receiving diminishing financial return and sensing a lack of focus in the work itself. In 1997 Alison determined to concentrate her work in her home town of Bentham and apply arts in health techniques to long-term community development there. She set up a charitable company, Pioneer Projects Ltd, to further that aim. Bentham is a small rural town that combines industrial production and craft traditions with agricultural activity. The town has a population of 3000 and a rural-area GP practice population closer to 8000.

Looking Well was envisioned as providing an informal community space where arts, health promotion and lifelong-learning programmes could come together in a setting designed to promote a positive disposition, build confidence and skills, and enable people to support each other and solve problems together. Domestic in feel, scale and furnishings, it offers a congenial space with the atmosphere of a well-functioning extended family developing supportive arts activities out of its own health needs assessments. It is cheap, simple and draws on local volunteer skills, and certainly at the level of community engagement it appears to work very effectively.

The community consultation that led to Looking Well being set up included a health needs assessment entitled *Getting Together*, commissioned by health and social care agencies in North Yorkshire in 1995.[15] Alison led a process of participatory information gathering and got local schoolchildren to interview elders in the town. The assessment focused on the specific health needs of a rural area with difficult-to-access health services.

In a traditionally conservative community, the arrival of a health project led by professional artists was met by some scepticism. Health professionals were keen to engage, however, and the community proved exceptionally responsive within a short period of time as acceptance and understanding grew. The very breadth of the approach may have been hard to grasp initially – how could work in the arts develop good health and positive attitudes? – but as its participatory ethos gained acceptance and momentum, those broad aims became embedded in the life of the centre.[16] In particular, its activities were seen to provide vital support and cohesion to the farming community during the 2001 foot-and-mouth crisis, and over time Looking Well has engaged with anything from the agricultural show to helping with funeral arrangements.

At Looking Well the concept of 'the artist' has never been confined to individual professionals; it is meant to encompass all those who wish to engage in creative production, developing new skills and often drawing on talents embedded in the communities themselves. This has resulted in work as diverse as a community garden, a rural towns' physical exercise project called Activate and health-themed events that are regenerating local traditions such as harvest festival, agricultural shows and carnival parades. Participation in Looking Well activities has developed beyond involvement in community events to the point where individuals have felt affirmed as artists and become keen to develop their technical skills and a more personal vision of what they want to build and achieve. Several participants have gone on to run workshops in the wider community, embracing a belief that engagement in creative process – whether it be creative writing or making large-scale processional lanterns – develops a sense of unity and engagement, offering purpose and fulfilment. For others, engagement with the work of the centre restored valuable patterns of work and self-belief.

Looking Well users include adults with mental health problems, cancer support groups, elderly people and vulnerable children and families, as well as many others who are drawn to activities through a more general sense of need or isolation. Within two years of its establishment in 1997 and with well over a thousand people using the centre, Looking Well achieved national recognition through receiving the King's Fund and SmithKline Beecham IMPACT Award for Excellence in Community Health. The facilities then expanded to include Looking Well Cottage, a space for complementary treatments, creative writing and self-help (and essential office space).

Buoyed by its success, in 2006 Looking Well raised funds to move from its rented premises to a specially renovated four-storey building. The new premises provide studios for artists and small creative enterprises, and there is an outdoor studio for larger-scale projects that may involve collaborative construction work. It sees its future role as facilitating the provision of training and mentoring programmes for artists wishing to engage with work in health and with health professionals who wish to develop artistic skills and perspectives.

The project has reached an exciting point in its development, where activities can now be perceived as much more influential upon mainstream thinking, which has changed significantly since Pioneer Projects began. It will likely continue to change and grow as an organisation motivated by individual energies and community needs rather than by policy-makers. Pioneer Projects is wary that centrally determined policy may not be the best driver of a local initiative.

Through Pioneer Projects and Looking Well, Bentham is known now for its annual harvest lantern procession and community bonfire, begun in 1997. There are several elements to the festivities. They may start in a small and discrete way with primary-school children celebrating harvest time by making fruit sculptures, lanterns, cards and gifts in workshops led by artists with parents and teachers. Others learn to play music and write songs for the occasion. They then walk in procession round the town with lanterns and music, taking gifts of small pots of jam made from local fruit to older and housebound people. All older people visited on the procession are personally contacted earlier in the week, providing an opportunity to identify any need and provide information and advice with back up from Age Concern and health workers. Then one week later, after more lantern-making workshops held in Looking Well, approximately 2000 people take part in a much larger lantern parade to the town's community bonfire, concluding with spectacular fireworks. Although the event relies on ticket sales and sponsorship in kind from local traders, in terms of effort it is very much Looking Well's gift to its community, establishing the goodwill profile that makes its year-round operations so accessible and successful.

It is evident that Looking Well has moved from being on the fringe of High Bentham, and thought by some to be 'alternative', to being now a central

organisation in the town, establishing these new traditions that cross generations. As well as partnering with health and social care services, the relationship
developed with High Bentham Primary School has been crucial, enabling the
school to build links between home and community. In an independent evaluation of Looking Well for the Lottery's New Opportunities Fund, the school's
(then) head teacher comments:

> Firstly, Looking Well has had a direct impact on the school curriculum through,
> for example, the lantern work and the performing arts work (shadow puppets)
> addressing social inclusion. When we looked at the social inclusion work we
> were aware of the need to target children exhibiting difficult behaviours and
> families becoming isolated in the community. The school and Looking Well
> together could do this; keeping an eye open. The work was intended to bring
> people back into the community. Because Looking Well focuses on the arts,
> it is practical, and helps teachers explore the different learning approaches
> of children. Some children learn best through practical application and
> Looking Well provides opportunity for that. The healthy school initiative was
> undertaken with Looking Well back-up. Now, children have bottles of water
> in the classroom, there's music in the classroom, and lots of cross-curriculum
> links have been made.
>
> Second, Looking Well's impact on the community is noticeable. Parent
> members of the PTA and parent helpers at the school refer to having been
> empowered by Looking Well. This has enabled us to pursue our work with
> parents to the extent that we now have an accredited training programme for
> parents in partnership with Craven College.
>
> Third, its impact on individual children and families is significant. Looking
> Well provides support for families in distress where the school is not able to do
> this. It provides such families with opportunities for friendship, networking and
> support. This is a very powerful tool. I can think of families who have turned
> around because of their involvement with Looking Well. I certainly will be
> heralding Looking Well as a key player helping to promote the health and well-
> being of Bentham kids in my report to Ofsted [the school inspectorate].[17]

Looking Well summarises its success in the following factors:
➤ it's adaptable
➤ it has the trust of the community
➤ it's not pie in the sky
➤ it's proactive in the community
➤ it's not burdened with committees
➤ it's not just a talking shop
➤ it reflects the needs of the community
➤ it's in the right sort of town – a mental health 'hot spot'.[18]

The Looking Well initiative has dared to think long-term and to nurture the personal development of its participants. Having now got the chemistry right in its partnerships with other agencies, it is going back to re-offering itself as an arts-led venture. Important to its lifecycle approach is engaging parents with children in all creative activities and connecting children with older people. The inclusive nature of the work and the space in which it evolves are crucial. The steady stream of visitors from primary care trusts and regeneration projects across the country is testament to the growing interest in seeding similar projects in other areas.

## CHICKENLEY 'ROOTS AND WINGS'

Mary Robson has travelled in a different direction from Alison to find the right context for embedding arts in community health, but she has likewise come to the view that the primary school environment must be the incubator of healthy emotional development and social integration in deprived and dysfunctional communities. Like Alison, she started out as a theatre designer and moved into participatory arts through Welfare State International, but she later developed a specialist pedagogic role in work with young people. Her focus has been largely on children at risk, assisting them to develop their understanding of emotions and responsibility through both creative and reflective practice.

Children's policy has never been so high on the public agenda. The UK government's Every Child Matters strategy, introduced in 2000, identified five national outcomes that all professionals working with children and young people needed to be working towards; these are being healthy, staying safe, enjoying and achieving, making a positive contribution and socioeconomic well-being.[19] The strategy provided a context through which to have joint conversations, joint planning and joint working by statutory and voluntary agencies, with clear processes to achieve those outcomes for children and young people. Crucially, they have had to involve children and young people in learning to take responsibility for achieving those outcomes for themselves. The National Children's Bureau has come to see the five outcomes as integrated rather than separate, and it has identified characteristics of good practice residing particularly in projects that foster creativity and emotional and social development. Such projects can ameliorate the process of transition, not only as it occurs in the school system but also possibly when a child undergoes difficult change and loss in his or her personal life.[20]

One such project, run by Mary Robson since 2003, is based at Chickenley Primary School in Dewsbury, Yorkshire. Chickenley is a socioeconomically deprived 'sink estate' on the outskirts of Dewsbury. Its primary school has had a troubled recent history. The school had a record of low academic achievement and uncommitted teaching staff – some children having experienced as many as 14 different class teachers in five years – so in 2001 it was taken into 'special measures' on the recommendation of the inspectorate. A dynamic new head teacher, Lesley Finnegan, was brought in to turn around the freefall in the school's reputation and improve its standards. However, she saw poor educational attainment in the context of a much wider social demoralisation and its impact on health. As she described it:

> I used to drive home in those first few weeks and think to myself, if this is mimicked across the country we are in serious trouble of losing people, people who are so damaged and challenged; especially children who need something to happen to improve their lives and their futures and the future of those communities. And that used to worry me because it was much more than being a head teacher in a school sorting out illiteracy and innumeracy.[21]

She reluctantly (because this could reinforce Chickenley's negative image) listed the problems that were both the cause and effect of her school's under-achievement as:
- ➤ low self-esteem/self-worth
- ➤ low attainment
- ➤ low staff morale
- ➤ low attendance
- ➤ poor home-school relationships
- ➤ poor attitude to learning
- ➤ poor behaviour
- ➤ poor reputation locally.

She then defined the moral purpose of her school to be:
- ➤ to raise aspirations and close the learning and performance gap between individuals – pupils, families and staff
- ➤ to treat everyone with respect but not compromise expectations
- ➤ to improve the physical environment of the school and of the community
- ➤ to encourage all to understand the big picture and their place in it.[22]

Lesley Finnegan sensed an alienation between the school and the community, manifest in parental antagonism and the children's lack of trust in their teachers:

> Learning didn't even come into it at that stage. But I wanted to engage their curiosity and develop belonging. The children needed to feel like they belonged somewhere. A big part of it is friendship and respect for individuality. We came across enormous challenges around friendship and transition because I was aware that our children were anxious about going on to high school. I saw this

as a long-term piece of work because Chickenley doesn't have a huge movement of its population; families stay, and so our children become our parents.[23]

She felt the problem could not be addressed simply through a revisionist approach addressing behaviour problems and attendance or through implementing a learning-improvement plan. She was looking for a nurturing approach to prevent children's mental ill health and stimulate appetite for learning. At a head teachers' conference in Manchester, she heard how an inner-city school there had recruited a parent who was a visual artist to work with children who were damaged both emotionally and socially – and this had also produced stunning visuals affirming the school's values. Lesley was fired up to achieve something similar, to be pitched on a more ambitious scale than a short-term arts in education project. She subsequently sought, and got, support from the Children's Fund to instigate a long-term school-based arts project, and through Loca, an arts and regeneration agency that was partnered with the Children's Fund, she and Mary Robson were introduced to each other.

Mary Robson and Lesley Finnegan found they had a strong rapport and a mutual interest in developing a project that would be informed by the work of

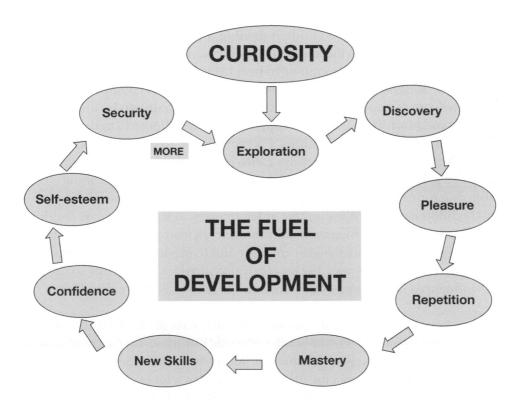

**FIGURE 4** The 'Curiosity' learning cycle

Bruce Perry, a Texas psychologist who works with children in trauma. Perry uses the 'curiosity sequence', which is prevalent in child development thinking, as it offers a simple, straightforward pathway for both delivery and evaluation.[24] Mary Robson adapted this sequence to her diagrammatic illustration of a desired learning cycle, which is reproduced here with her permission (*see* Figure 4).

In an initial meeting with school staff, it was explained that this idea about curiosity being 'the fuel of development' was going to underpin what they were about to do. Support artists were then recruited to programme an astonishing 70 person-days a term of specialist arts support. The artists and teaching staff have worked closely together on Roots and Wings, developing a programme of arts activity that includes the creation of new traditions to celebrate rites of passage and transition and the use of the arts to foster social and emotional development in children.[25] Many of the pupils live with violence – verbal, physical, emotional, domestic and media-delivered – on a daily basis. The children have been guided along a searching journey focusing on self, emotions, expression of emotions, and different ways to depict such complex messages through a range of art forms.

Roots and Wings puts children in the driving seat to help change some aspects of local culture, prevent mental ill health and set the scene for a more nurtured generation. A deeply held belief that an emphasis on unconditional positive regard will lead to children gaining a perceptive understanding of alternative ways of behaving and enhance their ability to learn pervades every nook of the project and is beginning to bear fruit. These children need different choices for adulthood, and some need better memories of childhood.

At the core of Roots and Wings is the art room, a space run by the children at break and lunchtimes with artist support. Children choose to make things of emotional content in these sessions. Encouragement to reflect on feelings has led to the children creating greetings cards, initially for friends and family but now also sold into craft outlets in the town, with the proceeds providing chari-table donations that the children determine. Sometimes there may be as many as 40 children in the art room, but order emerges in this bedlam as children assist each other in realising their art from concept to appraisal. It is not just an activity room; it is a space to foster empathy and to model and analyse relation-ships in a child-friendly way. The art room also provides a congenial space that has influenced the design of other areas in the school. As Mary describes it:

> We used to call it the studio, we now call it the art room because that's what the children term it. One of the first things we did was encourage the use of sofas in school. This is because at Southwick school in Sunderland the head introduced sofas and literacy went up; the reason being that a lot of children don't have comfortable furniture at home and more to the point they don't get to curl up on the sofa and read a book.[26]

The art room becomes the base for a 12-week summative art project by Year Six (top class) pupils. They explore self-portraiture containing depiction of their feelings and look to examples from their own lives and to art history for inspiration. These portraits are later exhibited and curated by the children in the local minster. Then in the last weeks of the summer term, they create large processional images expressive of the qualities and values they wish for themselves as they make their transition to high school next term. The children form their own carnival company, designating additional roles amongst each other for producing musical accompaniment, publicity and video documentation. Each year on the last Tuesday of summer term, the Year Six pupils parade up to the high school, followed by a growing number of parents and the cheers from the school gates of all the junior classes. The parade tableaux, whose structures are akin to the latticework of lanterns, have a richness of colour and exotic names such as 'The Waterfall of Wishes', 'The Rocky Mountains of Strength' and 'The Fearless Flames of Destiny'. When they arrive at the secondary school, Year Seven children are at the gates to greet them. A garland of origami birds on which each child has written a wish is presented to the head of the secondary when the Roots and Wings parade arrives, and the Chickenley head asks him, 'Will you please take care of our children? They are talented and special individuals.'

The resonance of this event is absorbed by all, revealing what the tradition and the ritual mean beyond the children themselves and where the adults are following them in terms of cultural change. As a parent said to Mary, 'My son came home and said, "The parade's coming up next week. I've got to be there and clap for them." And I said to him, "You clap, you cheer like you never have. You remember what it was like for you last year."'[27]

Within three years, the Roots and Wings programme significantly impacted on Chickenley Primary's performance at all levels. An Ofsted inspection report in May 2006 stated:

> One child wrote about her marvellous work of art, 'I think I am a painter now. I could work in a fast food restaurant, but being a painter is better'. Pupils are cherished as individuals. Education for personal and social health and citizenship is well organised to promote healthy and safe lifestyles. The initiative entitled *Roots and Wings* is an outstanding element which has raised the school's profile locally. Pupils' artistic skills, writing and personal development, for example, are enhanced by its many superb activities. Pupils who are talented in sports or the arts thrive on a curriculum which offers many worthwhile opportunities in these areas. This is reflected in their trusting attitudes and confident bearing.[28]

One inspector wrote to the children to say:

> We loved talking to you about the way that your school has improved in the last few years. The Roots and Wings project is marvellous. We particularly liked the art room and all that goes on in there.[29]

When adult visitors are taken by the children to view the self-portrait exhibition, they are frequently amazed by the children's insight not only into their own art but into that of their peers too. Mary attributes this to having reflective practice built in at every stage of the project. By this means, children are more confident to talk not only about what they do but also about what other people can do. The feedback from the children is that it gives them confidence hearing other people talk about their work as well.[30]

When Year Eight pupils in high school were asked of their memory of the art room, a common observation by them was that it was the one place in school where they could be sure not to be shouted at and where they would be listened to. The impact is also evidenced in the number of secondary school prizes awarded to former Chickenley pupils – two in 2005 and 34 in 2007 – and in the number of pupils from the estate electing to study art and design subjects for GCSEs.

Independent evaluation of the first three years of Roots and Wings used a combination of observation, self-assessment tools and interviews.[31] It endeavoured to record changes in children's development under three headings:

➤ improved educational attainment arising from better motivation, concentration and attendance
➤ improved ability to cope with challenges as a result of decision-making skills, assertiveness with peers and successful transition
➤ increased confidence from greater cooperation, contribution to teamwork and self-confidence.

The study found 'fields of outstanding impact' in confidence, motivation and concentration as regards the children's personal development. However, with the exception of art, it was not possible to find attributable impact on learning improvement in standard attainment tests. Most teachers, on the other hand, consider the art room to have had a significant effect on children's attitude and engagement throughout the school and curriculum, altering their own practice as a result towards sustaining a more empathic and positive approach to their learners. Mary remains pragmatic about the success:

> There is no magic wand. We don't start out with children who are really troubled and end up as model citizens after a few months because they do a bit of art. That's not what this is. This is ongoing, day to day, hour by hour, on your feet, thinking laterally and being driven by real care. Our 'sofa moments' happen not just between children but between staff as well. Like when a teacher comes

in to say 'It's a Monday morning. They are *more* tired and *more* hungry – not refreshed after a weekend. So much has happened in their lives. Someone is in tears. Many are running around and out of the room. They don't need a maths lesson at this point. They need someone to talk to about what they've been through. And I've got to talk to them about multiple numbers.' Teaching can be a very lonely and exacting profession, with people looking over your shoulder all the time. When I saw this teacher the next day I said, 'How are you doing?' and she said, 'I'm much better from that conversation we had.' The culture now allows for those conversations to happen, that it is alright to put your hand up and say, 'Enough, enough.' One of the things we are very keen to get going is reflective practice between staff too.[32]

There have been all manner of ancillary activities, such as getting the dinner ladies to read to the children during the annual Day of the Dictionaries, an event at which all children spend a day seeking and considering words and their meanings. Another offshoot is Game Plan, an innovative project that empowers Year Five children to explore and recognise personal aspirations and to examine issues of community: What is community? What do we get from community? What roles do people have in our community? A very enjoyable part of the project is a day when the school is visited by many professional people who all have different roles in life. These might include a firefighter, a vicar, a college lecturer, a professional rugby player and a shop manager, amongst many others. Opportunities arise for the children to ask the visitors what qualities they need to perform their role in society and what they enjoy about their role. The project also goes 'on the road', with children making visits to the local community. Trips include a 'fact-finding mission' to the University of Huddersfield so they can see where education leads. Once the children have collected the information, they are tasked with developing a board game that examines the decisions and dilemmas involved with the different roles within the community. The language acquisition focus from the Day of the Dictionaries combined with the modelling and scenario-building inherent to Game Plan is providing the children with appraisal skills that spill over into their classroom learning. The art room is influencing the style of teaching and the overall culture of the school.

To mark the halfway point in the school year and the coming of spring, lanterns have entered the iconography of Chickenley. Since 2005, an annual event known as Lanternland has taken place on a March evening. Rather than a procession, this is an installation in the school grounds in which each child's sculptural lantern is exhibited within a candlelit maze of pathways. The community gathers in the school hall for homemade soup and lantern songs, with children working the crowd as storytellers and then leading everyone out into the installation. The transformation is complete as photos are taken of families posing by lanterns. The dissemination of this event includes building international connections around it. When some visiting South African teachers took part in the event in 2008, they learned that the Chickenley children had raised almost £1000 from their greetings card sales to support arts development work in shack schools in Soweto.

Roots and Wings has directly influenced the development of arts in health programmes in several North East schools that CAHHM has brought together to share practice and research. Inspired by the Chickenley parade, one school in North Tyneside, Rockliffe Junior School, has developed its own transition event in the form of a feast for the Year Four class who are moving on to middle school. The feast is produced mostly from food grown by the children in the grounds. The class is treated to special table decorations made by the rest of the school, to souvenir crockery that they have made themselves and to a 'passing out' parade under a floral playground arch. Other ideas have emerged and been built into the project, including storytelling linked to the growing and watering of food, artist designed menu boards and year-round arts activity to stimulate children's eating choices. School catering services are also encouraged to participate.

Inspired by the Southwick parade, Tilery Primary School in Stockton-on-Tees is developing an annual lantern procession that reflects and celebrates the local area's transition to a multi-ethnic community, with a vigorous approach to raising health awareness. The event includes a spur procession of lanterns traversing a new pedestrian bridge over the Tees that connects Tilery's district with Durham University's Queens Campus. This event symbolically attests to the university's growing commitment to improving the health and prospects of its host community.

For me, 'the lantern road' has the characteristics of an anastomosis, defined as 'the connection of separate parts of a branching system to form a network, as of leaf veins, blood vessels, or a river and its branches'.[33] Already this 'road' is radiating and then converging through the case examples described in this and the previous three chapters – for example, through the exchange links that Mary is developing with CDP in Johannesburg and through Alison taking up the next Healthway fellowship in Western Australia to work with Christine Jeffries-Stokes, a paediatrician developing arts in health with indigenous communities in the goldfields territory. Mary has also been experimenting in recent years with different lantern designs – small globular ones that can be attached to children's pushchairs, buildings that can be transformed into giant lanterns by creating illuminated paper-cuts in all the windows, and electrically lit lanterns that you can run with. The phenomenon of lanterns is becoming the apogee of community arts practice – reflexive, inclusive and inventive – providing 'live' examples of social cohesion and offering collective artworks to a shared ideal of community health.

## REFERENCES

1 Williams R. *Towards 2000*. London: Chatto and Windus; 1983.

2 Fox J. *Eyes on Stalks*. London: Methuen; 2002. p. 75.

3 Jones A. *The Lantern Procession: past, present and future*. Ulverston: Welfare State International; 1987.

4 Lynch E, Robson M. *Lanterns '88*. Ulverston: Welfare State International; 1988.

5 White M. Resources for a journey of hope: the work of Welfare State International. *New Theatre Q*. 1988; **15**: 195–208.

6 Gateshead and South Tyneside Health Authority. *Report of the Director of Public Health 1992*. Gateshead: Gateshead and South Tyneside Health Authority; 1992.

7 Robson M. Happy Hearts. In: Kai J, Drinkwater C, editors. *Primary Care in Urban Disadvantaged Communities*. Oxford: Radcliffe Publishing; 2004. p. 154.

8 Ibid.

9 Robson M, White M. From ice to fire: arts in health for social inclusion. *Mailout*. 2003; June/July: 19–21.

10 Robson, op. cit. p. 155.

11 Robson, White, op. cit. p. 20.

12 Centre for Arts and Humanities in Health and Medicine. *Wrekenton's Happy Hearts Lanterns: 10th anniversary*. Durham: University of Durham (CAHHM); 2003.

13 Everitt A, Hamilton R, White M, editors. *Arts, Health and Community: a study of five arts in community health projects*. Durham: University of Durham (CAHHM); 2003.

14 Russell A, White M. *Making Sense: a report of the seminar at Cartwright Hall, Bradford, June 19–20, 2003*. Durham: University of Durham (CAHHM); 2003.

15 Craven Health Promotion. *Getting Together*. Yorkshire: Craven Health Promotion; 1995.

16 Jones A. Leading the way to healthy communities. *Mailout*. 2005; April/May: 6–7.

17 Everitt A. *Looking Well Evaluation*. Bentham: Pioneer Projects; 2003.

18 Ibid.

19 www.everychildmatters.gov.uk/strategy/ (accessed 5 August 2008).

20 Worthy A. *Spotlight Briefing: supporting children and young people through transition*. London: National Children's Bureau; 2005.

21 Finnegan L, Robson M. Unpublished transcript of presentation at Children's Fund Conference; 9 Nov 2005: Yorkshire; Dewsbury Minster.

22 Ibid.

23 Ibid.

24 Perry B. *Curiosity: the fuel of development*. Available at: http://teacher.scholastic.com/professional/bruceperry/curiosity.htm (accessed 5 August 2008).

25 Robson M, White M. The potent arts. *J Public Ment Health*. 2004; 6(4): 12–13.

26 Finnegan L, Robson M, op. cit.

27 Ibid.

28 Kirklees Education Authority. *Ofsted Inspection 282150*. Huddersfield: Kirklees Education Authority; 2006.

29 Ibid.

30 Cremin C. *Interim Evaluation of Roots and Wings*. Dewsbury: Chickenley School; 2008.

31 Raw A. *Chickenley Creative Kids Project: independent evaluation for year 3*. Dewsbury: Children's Fund; 2006.

32 Finnegan L, Robson M, op. cit.
33 Definition from The Free Dictionary. Available at: www.thefreedictionary.com/anastomosis (accessed 5 August 2008).

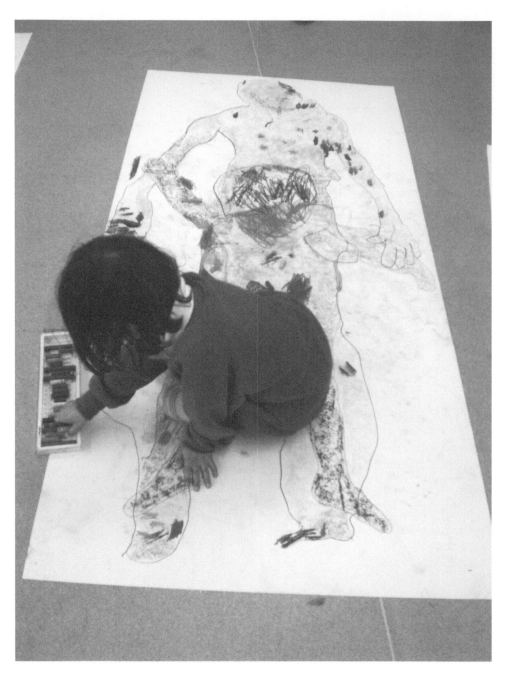

'My Little Flower': picturing the parent/child bond. PHOTO: MARY ROBSON

# CHAPTER 8

# The burden of proof . . . or the benefit of the doubt?

I feel a responsibility as a scientist who knows the great value of a satisfactory philosophy of ignorance, and the progress made possible by such a philosophy, progress which is the fruit of freedom of thought. [...] If you know that you are not sure, you have a chance to improve the situation.

Richard P. Feynman, *The Meaning of It All*[1]

The arts in community health field is now mature enough to analyse its mistakes in research and practice, and this means that honest appraisal with reflective practice is not a post-mortem on failure but rather, like good detective work, the process of elimination that may arrive at the truth.

To appreciate the challenge that arts in health poses to evaluation, it is important to acknowledge not only the unknown but also the unknowable. I am increasingly interested in the hidden meaning of arts in health, how some projects enable participants to go on a public and private journey and how there is often a resonance and communication going on that is not easily accessible to observers – such as the unannounced creation of memorial lanterns or the significance of the cultural mores of Zulu women in Siyazama, as reviewed earlier in the case examples. There is a lot we do not and cannot empirically know that is nevertheless an integral yet immeasurable part of the well-being experienced by the participants. The benefits of participation in arts in community health are to date only partly substantiated and so are also partly unknown. As Feynman suggests, however, this should not constrain the value of bringing a spirit of deep and meaningful inquiry to pioneering work.

Matarasso's landmark study *Use or Ornament?* on the social impact of participation in the arts noted rather inconclusively from its questionnaire survey that about half of those interviewed (48%) reported feeling better or healthier since becoming involved in the arts.[2] This was loosely attributed by participants to feelings of improved well-being rather than to a specific health benefit. As Michael Wilson has pointed out, 'It is difficult to describe what we mean by well-being without asking the question: what is health for?'[3] Another problem with well-being as an outcome of arts activity is that it too easily equates with well-meaning. It can appear woolly and congratulatory unless a guiding framework of evaluation is placed on the process of the activity itself. It is important, however, that this framework gives some credence to participants' assertions about feeling better, because that self-perception of improved vitality affirms that participants are at least not feeling worse, or the same, as the result of the activity.

Sometimes the pitch of an arts project can seem wrong to a health professional's perspective. A project can set a big goal such as improved well-being, but it also needs to demonstrate small things. This is not as obvious as it seems. Some years ago, I observed a dance project in London for people with obesity problems. The project's stated aim was to foster self-esteem and well-being in the participants, but it neglected to consider whether weight loss might be a measurable indicator of health gain from the activity. One should perhaps balance this easy criticism with the question of whether only looking for an instrumental benefit from the arts activity obscures its significance in having a transformational effect on participants. Participatory arts practice by its nature looks to do more than the obvious, and an open perspective is required in seeking its benefits. Participatory arts, as distinct from art therapy, does not focus directly on a health outcome; it aims to produce work of artistic quality through a mode of engagement that may also have beneficial social outcomes that can indirectly impact on health.

How can we better substantiate claims of improved well-being so that participants' testimony is not relegated to just anecdotal evidence? I think that to answer that question we need to see how value structures are formed from participatory arts activities and how they can impact on a social model of health. This also has bearing on an underlying question for me in this book as to how and why shared creativity may help construct a healthier community and what causal links can be established between the two. It would help if the articulation of value could be as worthy of attention as a demonstration of causality. As Robert Pirsig says in *Lila: an inquiry into morals* (the sequel to his 1970s cult travelogue *Zen and the Art of Motorcycle Maintenance*):

> To say that 'A causes B' or to say that 'B values pre-condition A' is to say the same thing. What appears to be an absolute cause is just a very consistent pattern of preferences. Therefore when you strike 'cause' from the language and

substitute 'value' you are not only replacing an empirically meaningless term with a meaningful one: you are using a term that is more appropriate to actual observation. The greatest benefit of this substitution of 'value' for 'causation' and 'substance' is that it allows an integration of physical science with other areas of experience . . . If science is a study of stable patterns of value, then cultural anthropology becomes a supremely scientific field. A culture can be defined as a network of social patterns of value.[4]

It is tempting to take this view, but I am not convinced that 'A causes B' and 'B values pre-condition A' is saying the same thing, because the former is in the realm of empiricism and the latter in the realm of metaphysics. A cultural anthropologist is likely to be an empathic evaluator, but Pirsig is wrong to declare their science is based on 'stable patterns of value', because he immediately confuses this with 'social patterns of value'. They are not the same thing either. Moreover, some cultures mutate and thrive while others are ossified by custom. As Picasso once said, 'tradition is about having a baby; not wearing your father's hat.'

Although Pirsig's declaration does not stand up as a quid pro quo substitution, it is an insightful recognition that the effect of a cultural construct cannot be reduced to linear causality. This has implications for how arts in health might be evaluated. Making progress in this has been confounded by an insistence on assessing art as a form of treatment – proving 'A causes B' – rather than as a way of viewing the world – revealing how 'B values pre-condition A'. Trying to fit into the treatment mode can deflect arts in community health projects from their inherent strengths.

This is a recurrent problem. In documenting and examining the creative processes in arts in community health (and those of the wider arts in social inclusion agenda), should we be tracking separately the indicators of therapeutic benefit and the revelatory impact of effective quality artwork? Or maybe it is better that they are seen as interfused, or one could end up with art therapy without its inherent discipline and the outcomes may be even harder to substantiate. The issue should be to understand the creative process better in order to generate better-quality art – but understanding what is revelatory in this can be more important than technical accomplishment. If arts interventions are to be pervasive and of quality, they will also on occasion be radical and challenging – to participants, to artists and to the sectors that support and fund them. It is inherent to the effectiveness of arts in health intervention that it is permitted, within safe and supportive parameters, to engage with the 'madness' of art and its making. By its very nature art pushes against barriers, boundaries and preconceptions, and its creative energy in promoting health and social inclusion may necessarily be volatile. This is why qualitative evidence from participants repeatedly affirms the felt experience of art as a counter to the circumstances and symptoms of ill health or social exclusion. An assessment of an arts in health project on Teesside noted that:

> As we have evaluated projects we have noted that there is a tension between the artistic and the social aims and objectives of the programme, which requires a much more open interpretation of the definition of quality, and suggests that a more useful focus could be on the value of the creative process.[5]

The most successful projects appear to be those that lay down a social pathway to channel awakened enthusiasms. But it is also important to consider what constitutes quality in the health environment, so consensus on quality needs to be found through dialogue with health professionals too.

Some studies focus specifically on arts in health and look for evidence of therapeutic benefit, while others take a broader perspective in attempting to identify a connection between cultural participation and well-being and how that impacts on individuals and their communities. The former type addresses a medical model of health, and the latter aims to influence social policy. Both approaches have been fraught with problems, but it is important first to establish what practitioners of arts in health hope to achieve from their activities. The arts have always done a great job of turning complexity into revelation, but artists who successfully engage with communities often do not do so well in evaluating the impact of their activity on them.

The race to capture an evidence base to support the ascendancy of practice in arts in community health can sometimes seem like a treadmill. CAHHM's review for the Health Development Agency of documents from arts in health projects concluded that the majority of practitioners in arts in community health recognise that it is important to evaluate their activity.[6] Many are attempting to do so, but they are struggling to find appropriate methods, and the evaluation they carry out is frequently inadequate. A serious and widespread shortcoming is a failure to state and agree clear aims for a project. There is uncertainty about what evaluation methods to use and what methods will be acceptable to other stakeholders. There is also concern that a requirement for quantitative evaluation will affect and damage the delivery of the work. In particular, there is concern about the requirements of medical practice. Whatever method of evaluation is adopted, practitioners can only collect appropriate data and evidence if they are clear about their aims and about what effect is intended.

The CAHHM review, undertaken by John Angus, looked at (mostly unpublished) evaluation reports and internal project assessments from over 150 arts in health projects in the UK. It concluded that evidence can be supplied simply to show that arts in health projects are addressing health and social participation, and this work can be described. It is more difficult to provide evidence that these projects have an effect on health, social exclusion and civic participation. There is not a lot of reliable evidence on the effects of arts in health projects, because it is not always clear what effects are intended.

Health may be expressed not only in the emotional and bodily engagement of participants in an arts activity but also in the ancillary benefits that can be tracked from this. With this holistic approach in mind, one national arts in mental health study looked at the personal development of participants as 'distance travelled' through the social process of engagement in communal creative activity.[7]

There are plenty of studies to review both in published and 'grey' literature, although literature reviews can inadvertently confuse our perception of the arts in health field, as they tend not to attempt a taxonomy of practice to match the diversity of contexts in which the studies were produced. In Rosalia Staricoff's evidence review of medical literature for Arts Council England,[8] for example, many of the cited reports are only indirectly relevant to arts practice, as they primarily concern art therapies and the effects of pre-recorded music on patients – indeed music predominates in the studies found. Staricoff acknowledges that a lot more research needs to be done on arts engagement with patients and on community-based approaches. She also recommends more research into the specific effects on health of individual art forms, and while this might reveal interesting correlations in specialist areas such as neurology and psycho-immunology, it could confine research to investigating art as a mode of treatment within a medical rather than social model of health.

The Arts Council England study *Your Health and the Arts*[9] followed on from Staricoff's literature review. This report acknowledges that most research on engagement in the arts does not include information on associations with health, and much of what has been reported is based on small-scale, locally based projects. *Your Health and the Arts'* findings, however, are based on a survey of over 12 000 people carried out by the Office for National Statistics. Of these people, 85% had attended an arts/cultural event in the previous year, 60% had attended a film, 46% had attended a library, 27% had attended a carnival and 25% had attended a drama. The key finding is that those who attend artistic events are more likely than others to report good health, even when other variables such as income and age are taken into account, and 'participants were more likely than non-participants to regard themselves as having very good or good health (overall 81% as compared with 69%). The differences were most significant for sociable activities (84% compared with 73%).'[10] This helps corroborate findings from a longitudinal study in Scandinavia by Umeå University, which noted lower mortality rate in arts attendees over a 10-year period.[11]

Further quantitative research from Healthway in Western Australia provides longitudinal survey data that correlates arts attendances with health and lifestyle profile.[12] (Perhaps this could become a norm of national arts councils' statistical research and thereby reinforce the health connection?) Healthway's research confirms that state-wide audiences for arts events have incrementally increased since the early 1990s, that more females than males attend and that audiences in metropolitan areas are more frequent attendees than are audiences in country areas. More interestingly, it also reveals that arts attendees have a more balanced diet and are less likely to smoke and that over 40% have personal involvement in an arts activity. Healthway has used this data to calculate, through a cognitive behaviour change model, the impact of its sponsorship of arts events in encouraging lifestyle change. This has shown the health messaging to have achieved 'awareness' at 71.8%, decreasing through 'comprehension', 'acceptance' and 'intention' to 'motivated action' at 10.7%. Success requires a high initial score on 'awareness' in order to achieve the commitment to behaviour change.[13]

## SEEKING GOOD QUALITATIVE EVIDENCE

Quantitative evidence so far has provided some broad factual brushstrokes about the correlation of arts consumption and health awareness, but understanding the actual engagement process of arts in community health requires more complex qualitative study. It needs to be recognised that there are crucial misunderstandings around the aims, intentions and evidence for arts in health activity, and there is often a mismatch between the aims of the practitioners and the expectations of those requesting the evidence. The practitioners are addressing a wide range of particular circumstances in many ways and with a wide range of assumptions. Those requesting evidence seem to be expecting effects on individual health and behaviour, but they are not stating that explicitly. A similar problem has emerged in Australia, as Christine Putland of Flinders University succinctly observes:

> Evidence is said to remain elusive despite the proliferation of initiatives and government investment. Responses to this issue can broadly be characterized as health perspectives (calling for more scientific approaches to evaluation research that go beyond anecdote and opinion) and arts perspectives (concerned about reductive measures and narrowly prescribed social outcomes).[14]

In order to make progress in this search for evidence, it is essential that all parties clarify their intentions, assumptions and requirements. The practitioners need to state clearly what they are aiming to achieve. The funders and others requesting evidence need to state clearly for what effects they require evidence and what would be acceptable as evidence. Then better evaluation tools need to be devised and tested; these tools need to be sensitive to the processes of the work but also robust enough to delineate outcomes. There are indications that much more evidence is available but it needs to be dug out. It may be that NHS trusts and other agencies, accustomed to management and evaluation protocols, assume that collected evidence can be readily presented.

It would appear that the arts in community health field has been caught in a bind. Unless it produces a more rigorous evidence base for its work, it will not gain access to better sources of funding from the health sector, and because it does not have access to sufficient funding, it is struggling to work up this evidence base.[15] The bind tightens when arts in community health projects attempt to approach evaluation of their work in a way that satisfies the health sector's view of what constitutes appropriate evidence. Before attempting to unlock this dilemma, a degree of realism is required. Until recently, with the development of larger 'cluster' programmes, the practice has been small-scale, local and poorly resourced, although fuelled by deeply committed artists and involved healthcare professionals using their best efforts to gather indicative evidence from participants about whether there are any social, educational and health benefits and, if there are, what is their nature and extent.

Because of the wide range of potential benefits, the questions that arts in community health can pose for research are complex. This kind of creative intervention is attempting to do two things at once: to convey the therapeutic benefits for individuals from participating in arts activity and to convey the value of collective creativity in helping to build social cohesion for a healthier community. Such an interweaving of objectives seems to me to be valuable at a time when health promotion approaches are becoming polarised between informed choice and coercion.

The rationale and practice of cross-sector development in arts in community health needs to focus on clusters of demonstration projects. CAHHM's literature review of arts and adult mental health for the UK government's Social Exclusion Unit identified several projects built up through local cross-sector partnerships that could usefully collaborate in such a programme.[16] If the arts in community health field could, as a collective body, agree on the common aims and issues, agree on a way of evaluating and then share and collate the results, the field would achieve a critical mass of information. To get this critical mass, there needs to be joint funding applications for research-guided practice by like-minded organisations. This research, and the projects concerned, must be longer-term in order for them to be able to achieve effects and for them to be evaluated effectively. In conjunction, to combat the stress and emotional challenges that often accompany their work, artists could benefit from the professional supervision that is a norm of art therapy practice. Should this also be offered to other professionals in the arts in health field – not just artists – it would serve the additional purposes of building reflective practice into projects as a basis for evaluation and strengthening the fundamental relationships that underpin the work.

To determine exactly how, not just whether, participatory arts can impact on health, it is important to redress not only gaps in evidence but also gaps in practice. The arts in community health field would benefit from more shared practice, training and equitable support from the arts funding system for arts projects in healthcare institutions and community-based ventures. Then research can take the form of comparative case studies, pooling data to construct larger and more robust samples for quantitative survey and assessing the suitability of certain projects to attempt randomised control trials (RCTs).

An immediate call for more refined experimental approaches such as RCTs is premature relative to the capacity and experience of the sector and the wide range of factors that would need to be accommodated for sensitive and robust evaluation. Tom Smith argues the need first to distinguish between research and evaluation and to undertake the former as a means to provide a framework for collection of evidence. He cautions on designing randomised control trials:

> It has been suggested that the impact claimed from arts/health projects should be exposed to randomised control trials. In time, this may be the case. Research into at least two dimensions – those that claim therapeutic impact and support-ive effects on health provision – may generate hypotheses that RCTs could test. However, there are two main problems in suggesting that arts/health should be tested in this way. First, RCTs are essentially evaluative, and hypotheses are still to be developed. Secondly, it is questionable how sensitive and respectful RCTs are to concepts that are marginal to science: subjective, emotional and social elements of health.[17]

Recent studies indicate there has been a welcome shift to conducting rigorous evaluations of community-based arts interventions within a social model of health, rather than pushing them into a clinical model where the 'gold standard' of RCTs seems inappropriate for the inherent complexity and numerous variables involved in arts in community health. This is not a cop-out; it reflects serious enquiry by arts and social science disciplines in order to understand possible connections between creativity, health and citizenship.

Carolyn Kagan of the Research Institute for Health and Social Change at Manchester Metropolitan University, who evaluated the second phase of the Pathways project I referred to in Chapter 3, sums up well the challenges to evaluating sensitively the complexities inherent in arts in community health:

> The consensus (both common sense and evidence based) is that art has a positive impact on health. But this begs the question of what 'positive impact' and 'health' are. Some forms of art may have a clear physiological benefit (music, for example), others more of a psychological impact, and others a social impact (as in the Bromley by Bow example). Education for public health gain has rightly been considered a priority and I would agree the arts have a role

there. Importantly, a broader public health role might be expanded in terms of participative arts for those at health risk. Broad approaches to health include wellbeing as a vital part. This in turn must be seen as beyond happiness and satisfaction. So, the challenges of participating in art, the development of identity as 'artist' – often in the context of there being few identity spaces available for people – become important benefits. Even if physical or mental health does not improve, its deterioration may be prevented through participation in art. One of the tricky things is to identify who will benefit most from what kinds of art participation, and what are the qualities of an artist that are important in this work. I don't think we should shy away from asking these questions. When asking these questions we must be mindful of the raft of methodologies available to us in investigation. One priority in the health field must be to continue to challenge the hegemonic grip that positivism has over acceptable evidence. Different methodologies will be needed to capture the experiential gains of participating in art.[18]

In CAHHM's studies and in others, much qualitative evidence of benefit has been gathered, to a point where anecdotal evidence from participants is becoming moving and valid testimony. What constitutes valid and effective quantitative evidence still needs to be determined. No systematic review appears to have been undertaken yet of the social, clinical and cost benefits of participation in arts in health programmes. (Progress has been made, however, on some meta-analyses in the arts therapies field in the US.)[19] There is not much quantitative evidence, even with small samples, and little cost-comparison analysis with other interventions. No formal longitudinal study has been undertaken, although some projects based in healthcare settings have attempted to track clients' progress during term of treatment, post-discharge and (in some cases) readmission.

To help advance research in arts in community health, what happens outside formal evaluation of practice is still vitally important, and projects should devise their own checklists for ongoing assessment. Arts Council England's *Sharing Practice* by Gerri Moriarty[20] is not only a good practical manual for self-evaluation but also a welcome sign that the arts funding system is moving towards assisting more sophisticated evaluation. Many arts in health organisations are already thinking strategically as they develop their partnerships at local or sub-regional level, and they are shaping up the research questions that increasingly inform their work. Just as schools under their Ofsted inspectorate can be assessed for their 'ethos', arts in community health projects could be similarly reviewed. CAHHM's in-depth study of five community-based arts in health projects, described in Chapter 3, assessed the qualities and conditions that make for a strong ethos for projects.[21]

## TROUBLE SHARED IS TROUBLE HALVED?

It is good to know we are not alone. The complexities that challenge the evaluation of arts in community health are similar to those being wrestled with by programmes in public health and socioeconomic regeneration, where addressing health inequalities is closely connected with health improvement but the effectiveness of preventative strategy is difficult to assess as there are so many variables. Many in the field feel that assessment needs to move to a whole system approach, and central to this is how to understand and measure empowerment.

A literature review for the World Health Organization recognises the numerous variables and unpredictable outcomes for evaluation of empowerment and considers that traditional approaches are inappropriate because 'causal relationships may be too complex to uncover within a changing social environment.'[22] It notes that few studies explicitly test the effect of empowerment on health improvement, but the WHO sees such testing as a necessary prerequisite for measuring health gain. The WHO's literature review reveals that participation, psychological empowerment and sense of community can be best developed by strategies that build on the existing sense of community and cultural networks, and it calls for comparative design evaluation. It may be best not to rush into this, however, because 'empowerment' has become a loosely defined term in community development and is fraught with dilemma. In *Participation: the new tyranny*, Paul Francis argues that participatory approaches characterised by concern for sustainability, relevance and empowerment can still be an abuse of power and that simplistic notions are too readily made about 'the community'.[23]

It may be helpful to look first at how recent large-scale community regeneration initiatives with a strong health component have been assessed. The King's Fund publication *Finding Out What Works* is a useful analysis of complex community-based initiatives such as Health Action Zones, New Deal for Communities and Neighbourhood Renewal.[24] It sees that the underlying issue for effective evaluation and evidence generation is the creation of a learning culture through knowledge-building and network development. These initiatives are hard to evaluate because of their size and the speed with which they are rolled out and because they are trying to address multiple problems within shifting political environments. The report says there is not yet a proper learning culture for this, and RCTs would be difficult to apply. Evaluators inevitably cannot be objective, and 'theory of change' models may be the way forward with participatory evaluation. I am reminded of Common Knowledge when the study states that 'Overall it seems helpful to focus on knowledge-building, rather than merely promoting evidence-based policy and practice. However, this will require a synthesis of radically different cultures and philosophies about how people and organisations learn and change.'[25]

The report perceives a tension between the political demand for 'quick wins' and a longitudinal 'theory of change' approach that involves on-the-ground partners in the research. A shared understanding of standards is also required in research design. It argues that these big initiatives to tackle health inequalities have not really been based on evidence but on hunches and that they were selective of the outcomes of previous research to support their case.

*Finding Out What Works* argues that RCTs can only work if built in from the outset. A more process-oriented approach is called for, but there has been a lack of capacity in this to interpret and disseminate evidence. Furthermore, evidence-based working restricts risk-taking and innovation, so contradictions then arise with encouraging 'blue skies' thinking. The study senses a shift in government thinking towards recognising the complexity of participatory evaluation as large programmes produce a plethora of overlapping stories rather than definitive findings. It notes that 'a complex view of change pays more attention to history, culture and relationships, and sees change emerging from whole systems as they evolve over time'.[26] Ignoring this may be why some health action zones faltered when primary care trusts took them over and channelled their activity primarily into smoking cessation schemes.

Taking a complex view of change requires a qualitative analysis that is more rigorous than the anecdotal testimony that has so far constituted most evaluation of art in community health. It has been argued that qualitative research does not dismiss anecdotal testimony out-of-hand, because it attempts to ground and test it within the real-life circumstances of participants' experiences.[27] Although the principles that constitute this form of action-based research are intellectually acceptable in the social sciences field, they do not attain the 'gold standard' required of evidence-based medicine.

I see that the problem lies not so much with the method as with the desired audience for arts in health research, because the positivism of medical science seems less ready to accept holistic forms of explanation, preferring the presentation of individual pathology. Because crucial decisions have to be made on that presentation, success is predicated on short-term beneficial treatment of individuals rather than on the complex evolution of a social cure. Arts in health has unfortunately tended to vacillate between medical and social models of health in attempting to prove its efficacy. In the field of medical humanities, however, the 'interpretivist' approach is seen to have practical application to the patient consultation and to wider social malaise. It is not only a means of evaluation but also a medium for ascertaining a diagnosis that connects individuals' illnesses with their whole selves and their social circumstances.

The psychological dimension of narrative-based medicine brings a contextual relevance to the identification of symptoms and appropriate treatment, but this can also produce difficulty for itself. As psychologist John Launer observes, 'There is the cultural position of psychiatry itself, in an uncomfortable no-man's land between conventional medical science and a search for meaning which extends into political and religious domains . . . psychiatry is the only area of specialist medicine where talking and listening are explicitly understood to be therapeutic.'[28] This 'no-man's land' can create a similarly uncomfortable situation for arts in health in attempting to prove empirically the benefits of empathic communication from the collection of anecdotal testimony. I am reminded of Richard Smith's *British Medical Journal* editorial about health as 'adaptation, understanding and acceptance'.[29] If health might be conceived in the psychological domain as a search for meaning, then reflective practice and art's search for value can be important adjuncts in the quest for this.

## WHERE TO BEGIN

In terms of developing a case for government funding based on evidence, arts in community health is still in the early stage of the appraisal and evaluation cycle as set out in the Treasury *Green Book*,[30] somewhere between the rationale and the setting of objectives. (This may be true of the arts in health field as a whole.) But as the Cabinet Office Strategy Unit's *Creating Public Value* report has noted, the weakness to date in the 'new public management' model has been that 'Those things that were easy to measure tended to become objectives and those that couldn't were downplayed or ignored.'[31] Educationalist Gerald Lidstone also cited this at an ippr seminar on education and social inclusion, noting that 'a robust analysis is fine, but that it should be conducted in the same manner as an economic appraisal is maybe to miss the point.'[32] The user's voice in arts in health work is central to its evaluation, and it requires a sophisticated assessment of qualitative evidence rather than short-cut analysis of cost efficiency alone. Lidstone also drew attention to a report by the Council for Museums, Archives and Libraries[33] that has reworked the learning outcomes developed by the Quality Assurance Agency and applied them to assessing the impact of learning in museums. The five key headings (knowledge, skills, values, creativity and behaviour) could be further adapted to provide a suitable framework for assessing learning within arts in community health projects. It could ensure that developments in both practice and evaluation by arts in education and arts in community health projects are in dialogue within Arts Council England's social inclusion portfolio.

Crucial to exploring the link between arts and health as a social process is a more precise understanding of the holistic factors that contribute to well-being. The World Health Organization's Quality Of Life group (WHOQOL) has 15 research centres across the world independently contributing items to the development of a questionnaire derived from focus-group discussions with local respondents.[34] Questionnaire trials in each country then led to a 100-item scale reflecting four domains and 24 facets of quality of life, as summarised in the table below (*see* Table 1). I have here reversed the sequential order of the domains, as this seems better to reflect the process that an arts in health project goes through in assisting the creation of suitable environmental and social conditions for arts activity that may promote improvement in psychological and physical health with measurable outcomes. What I see as the most relevant facets for arts in health intervention have been highlighted in italics.

**TABLE 1** WHOQOL-100 facets and domains

| Domain | Facets incorporated within domains |
|---|---|
| Environment | • Financial resources |
| | • Freedom, physical safety and security |
| | • *Health and social care: accessibility and quality* |
| | • Home environment |
| | • *Opportunities for acquiring new information and skills* |
| | • *Participation in and opportunities for recreation/leisure activities* |
| | • Physical environment (pollution, traffic, noise, climate) |
| | • Transport |
| Social relationships | • *Personal relationships* |
| | • *Social support* |
| | • Sexual activity |
| Psychological | • *Bodily image and appearance* |
| | • *Negative feelings* |
| | • *Positive feelings* |
| | • *Self-esteem* |
| | • *Spirituality, religion, personal beliefs* |
| | • *Thinking, learning, memory, concentration* |
| Physical health | • *Activities of daily living* |
| | • *Dependence on medicinal substances and medical aids* |
| | • *Energy and fatigue* |
| | • Mobility |
| | • Pain and discomfort |
| | • Sleep and rest |
| | • *Work capacity* |

In WHOQOL's 'Environment' domain, arts could be seen to contribute to opportunities for acquiring skills and to participation in leisure activities. In the 'Social relationships' domain, arts in community health characteristically build personal relationships and provide social support. There is certainly qualitative evidence to posit that arts address all factors in the 'Psychological' domain, and this in turn suggests what benefits should be sought in the 'Physical health' domain. There would most likely be problems in reliable attribution of the health benefits to arts, but at least it focuses attention on specific outcomes. Understanding a positive role for arts in the 'psychological' domain might also encourage arts organisations themselves to administer simpler evaluation instruments, such as the Warwick-Edinburgh Mental Well-being Scale.[35]

One evaluation model with potential to adapt to arts in mental health projects could be the CORE (Clinical Outcomes in Routine Evaluation) System.[36] CORE has been designed in the UK for use in psychotherapy and counselling to measure outcome and provide for service audit, evaluation and performance management. It aims to answer the increasing demand in health sectors for evidence of service quality and effectiveness. It has the benefits of being free and easy to use, and it provides ongoing research and support services, including a benchmark club. CORE currently lacks information specific to the arts, but it is designed as a 'hub' onto which other sectors can develop standardised 'spokes' to collect sector- or population-specific information that complements the generic clinical and governance-oriented hub. The structure is such that an arts 'spoke' could attract cross-sector dialogue and assessment of its effectiveness.

The CORE evaluation model can prove an effective means of assessing reductions in medication and treatment/therapy requirements, against which cost-savings indicators might be attempted. Given there is some reticence among arts in health practitioners to attempt RCTs without further research, what might prove influential in the short term on health services and government decision-makers would be the identification of cost-savings indicators attributable to arts in health interventions. So CORE may be suitable for a specialist area of arts in mental health, and one major recent study has used it satisfactorily as a measurement tool.[37] Generally, however, it seems fair to say that as the practice of arts in community health is in its infancy, the appropriate methodologies for assessing it are still in incubation.

In Chapter 1 I mentioned that the Health Education Authority (HEA) report[38] into arts in health had identified three emergent approaches to evaluation, and I cite examples of these in the references:

1 *health-based approaches* testing what the arts contribute to self-esteem and its effect on qualitative self-assessments of well-being[39]
2 *sociocultural approaches* derived from recent assessments of the social impact of the arts[40]
3 *community-based approaches* adapted from social capital theory on health improvement.[41]

Each of these approaches can find some common ground in cultural interventions to address social inclusion. The challenge in research terms is to devise an appropriate and realistic evaluation design that can assess a range of potential outcomes encompassing therapeutic improvement, social inclusion and empowerment, mirroring the three approaches to evaluation identified in the

HEA report. While it is sometimes possible to classify an arts in health project under one of these approaches, in many cases you find that two or all three approaches are intertwined. A recent national study in the UK has evaluated arts and mental health projects that are using these combined approaches in an attempt to identify both health and social outcomes.[42] Importantly, the projects chosen for this study responded to a common evaluation framework and measures. However, the results are problematic in some key areas, as I shall explain later.

There are approaches in other fields that could be adapted. Influential sociological research by Ray Pawson and Nicholas Tilley[43] has described realistic strategies for complex community initiatives as requiring an understanding of context, mechanisms and intended outcomes, and this would certainly apply to participatory research in arts in community health. Emphasis here is placed on harnessing the insider knowledge of stakeholders as well as other sources of information and evidence. In the education sector, Shirley Brice-Heath, who has evaluated Arts Council England's Creative Partnerships initiative,[44] has advocated longitudinal ethnographic study that focuses on developments in the language skills of participants as both the measure and means of participatory evaluation.[45] These approaches are reliant on close engagement and effective partnership working and can be costly in terms of time.

Many arts in health projects aim to foster citizenship and provide a practical example of how to manifest public value, which is increasingly a driver of government policy. It is in this public value context that some recent studies have attempted to assess the impact of cultural services on social inclusion and well-being. In 2000 the Department for Culture, Media and Sport commissioned a study from the Centre for Leisure and Sport Research at Leeds Metropolitan University into the role of arts and sports in addressing social inclusion.[46] It selected 14 projects from across the country: three from sport, three from heritage, two from outdoor pursuits and six from arts and media. Two of the latter are arts in health projects: Common Knowledge in Tyne and Wear Health Action Zone and Walsall Council's arts in health programme. The report found that:

> there is little effective evaluation against social inclusion outcomes
> projects are more concerned to demonstrate they are delivering services than to engage in the complexities of evaluation
> far too little money has been invested in the evaluation process (unlike in the Sure Start programme of under-fives care or in Home Office measures to combat crime)
> there is a lack of clarity of outcomes and what they constitute
> participatory projects provide the basis of a cohesiveness that is of collective social benefit, but they have little success in opening up wider decision-making processes

➤ outcomes require longitudinal research to assess them
➤ project workers and participants must be integrally involved in any future research.

Regarding the impact of community-based cultural projects on health, the report concludes:

> There is evidence of cultural projects promoting health networks and increasing referrals to health services. Such health data needs to be collected systematically . . . The impact of these projects may be on a fairly small scale but they have been working with 'hard to reach' groups who had previously been left largely untouched by the health services. Their engagement offers the prospect not just of better health for them but also of lessening future costs of treatment.[47]

In government there has been growing interest in establishing whether there is connection between cultural participation and well-being. In Scotland, the Scottish Executive declared its belief in the value of arts to healthcare, and, while it may have put the cart before the horse, in 2005 it commissioned extensive and objective research into culture and well-being from the Centre for Cultural Policy Research at the University of Glasgow. This concluded that there may be an association between culture and well-being but that causal links are not yet determined, so the challenge is for policy to set realistic goals. The researchers' report, *Quality of Life and Well-being*,[48] reviewed 244 texts and found:
➤ while the evidence suggests an association between cultural and sports participation and an improved quality of life, there is no evidence of a causal relationship
➤ there is the *theoretical* possibility of a link between social connectedness, participation in culture and/or sport and quality of life, but conclusions have to be interpreted with care
➤ a linked issue is the question of the quality of the cultural and sport intervention and how far it has a bearing on outcomes
➤ there is no definitive set of indicators that can measure the contribution of culture and sport to quality of life and well-being
➤ underpinning any approach to the development of indicators is the issue of the policy goal: why does the public purse fund sports and cultural activity and to what end?

There is some degree of academic 'fence-sitting' in these conclusions. They see the resolution of a chicken-and-egg dilemma as being in the hands of the policy-makers. In my experience, policy-makers tend to see an unresolved evidence question as an excuse to stall for time rather than as a motivation. Yet if there is an apparent association between cultural participation and quality of life, the pointer is surely towards more field research to determine why that should be.

I now want to review some methodological approaches and techniques aiming to assist the development and assessment of arts in community health.

## USING LOG FRAMES AND PERFORMANCE INDICATORS

A study for CAHHM[49] that observed five community-based arts in health projects from 2000–02 recognised that artists, agency partners and participants can help by together closely tracking the evolution of a project and measuring it against its objectives, while allowing for unpredictable outcomes such as the degree of befriending that can take place between project participants. To assist this process, Angela Everitt introduced the methodology of log frames, or logical framework planning (*see* Table 2).

**TABLE 2** A matrix for logical framework planning

| Narrative | Indicators of effectiveness | Methods of verification | Assumptions/ risks |
|---|---|---|---|
| Goal | | | |
| Objectives | | | |
| Activities | | | |
| Inputs | | | |

A log frame has four columns and four rows. The first column, the Narrative of the project, sets out the overall goal, the objectives that should ensure that the project travels in the direction of this goal, the activities that will help meet the objectives and the inputs or resources needed to conduct these activities. It has an 'if-then' logic: if these inputs are secured, then these activities will be undertaken, then these objectives will be met, then this goal becomes realisable.

The second column, Indicators of effectiveness, addresses the question 'What would show us that we have been, and the extent to which we have been, successful in:

➤ getting nearer to realising our goal?

➤ going some way to achieving our objectives?

➤ undertaking our activities?

➤ securing the resources needed?'

The 'if-then' logic is continued both vertically and horizontally.

The third column, Methods of verification, addresses the question 'How will we discover those things that would show us that we have been successful?' Again, the 'if-then' logic is pursued vertically and horizontally.

The fourth column, Assumptions/risks, addresses those concerns that are summed up by the phrase 'but what if . . .?' This column allows us to identify those factors that may affect the project's pursuing the programme as identified in the other three columns. This column helps to build realism into the project, to develop understanding of risks and to identify factors critical to success. Some of these factors are outside of our control. Others alert us to the need to be vigilant or to introduce additional activities to address factors potentially detrimental to the project.

Log frames are useful for project planning and management generally as well as for evaluation design. For evaluation, the second and third columns particularly help to ensure that monitoring, review and evaluation are built into the project. Log frames also help to accommodate the sometimes-different evaluation requirements of different stakeholders.

The log frame approach is largely derived from work in developing countries on an evaluation method known as participatory rural appraisal (PRA).[50] Its maxims are 'use your own judgement', 'play', 'embrace error' and 'relax', and it emphasises a learning framework, good rapport, non-professionalism and the use of non-verbal illustrations. PRA looks at differences rather than measurements and highlights the off-the-wall occurrences. A log frame, however, is labour-intensive to maintain, and its accumulation of process data on the narrative of a project can obfuscate clear measurement of change.

In *Participation: the new tyranny*, Paul Francis compares PRA with shamanism for its moral authority and belief in transformational learning, what he terms a kind of 'neo-animism' in the researcher's immersion in 'community', which he feels can stifle real debate: 'The key to behavioural change is seen to be as much a shift in the imagination as the generation of a new set of methods, rules and guidelines.'[51] Looking at the use of PRA by the World Bank in its social development projects, he concludes that 'the "social" is primarily interpreted in terms of process, consultation and partnership. Little attention is given to the underlying structural determinants of well-being',[52] and so therefore social-impact monitoring is weak and under-evaluated. Francis is provocative in seeing the weakness of calling for a change in imagination, particularly as it may be proffered as being somehow both method and proof. Does arts in community health practice have to take criticism like this on the chin, or is there a response we can make? What about continual reflective practice and long-term engagement mitigating the adverse elements of PRA? Is the origin of the criticism really just Francis' cynicism about the principles and values of PRA, which can be corrupted like any principles? What difference would it make within PRA if the focus was actually on improving well-being and not just on consultation? Francis poses challenging questions that need to inform the framing of research in future.

A programme in Melbourne, Australia, has used a log frame evaluation methodology in assessing a cluster of VicHealth-funded projects known as the Community Arts Development Scheme (CADS).[53] Its tabulation method also deployed a qualitative measure termed 'most significant change'. This gathered stories and reflections from participants at regular intervals and then selected the best of them (as commonly agreed) to go into a categories grid reflecting the main aims and themes of the project. While this does not constitute academically rigorous evaluation, I think it is a good attempt to get to the core meaning of a project from participants' perspectives.

A basic down-to-earth approach to evaluation could be the creation of a set of performance indicators (PIs) for an arts in community health project.[54] It is an (ideally) simple method of being able to assess the performance of a project at a given time. It does require, however, an agreement between all parties on what the indicators should be, along with close monitoring and regular review. PIs are commonly used in both health services and local authority arts departments, and they can be flexible to accommodate both quantitative and qualitative results. Importantly, they keep a project focused on its aims and objectives. A more ambitious project could combine PIs with a logistical framework planning approach as outlined above. Both require stakeholder involvement throughout and together can accommodate a larger holistic evaluation strategy. Some PIs may be project specific and others may be generic and applicable to other situations.

A performance indicator model has the virtue of simplicity in focus, but it has to be recognised that it can only be an aspect of a larger evaluation strategy. As Matarasso notes, 'what matters is performance in context',[55] and that context is shaped by stakeholders and project participants having an equal role in a five-stage process of planning, setting indicators, execution, assessment and reporting. If a project aims to achieve a process of change in a community, it is essential to have the informed consent of all involved and the opportunity to define and assess collectively the values that the activity aims to produce. Matarasso sees the process as not so much cyclical as spiral, with the final reporting stage setting out the next stage of a sustainable programme.

In addition, a project needs to gather evidence of quality in the arts activity, and because this is so subjective, Matarasso suggests following processes similar to market research. I can see that if this spiral progression were achieved, the quality assessment could feed into the social marketing approach currently being adopted in public health interventions. Demonstrating value in the quality of the art produced, and not just achieving performance indicators, is key to the dissemination of meaningful evidence. As the testimony of participants in successful arts in community health projects has consistently shown, a captured imagination has the power of conversion – but this can lead to over-exaggerated claims.

## MODELS OF TRANSFORMATION

There have been some recent evaluations that ambitiously attempt to demonstrate the process of acquisition of well-being by participants in community-based arts in health projects. The final report in 2008 on the three-year Invest to Save project of the Arts for Health unit at Manchester Metropolitan University[56] presents real insight into practice, which I think is lacking in many evaluations, but it is problematic in its findings. There were six projects chosen for in-depth study in this Treasury-funded programme: these covered mental health (Salford and Pendle Arts on Prescription schemes), older people (Stockport Arts and Health and Wearpurple Arts in Cheshire) and health culture and environments (Alder Hey Hospital Arts Project and LIME). The Invest to Save researchers used appreciative enquiry techniques to 'discover what is, dream what might be, design change and find destiny/destination'. Two kinds of well-being were identified: that which is hedonic (feels good) and that which is eudemonic (incites change).[57] The communal reflection days, which were central to the evaluation, aimed to assess people's confidence in both the approach and process. In a session I attended at Alder Hey, health staff participants spoke of how provocation about producing meaningful evidence is making evaluation more important and better. They felt that the transient effects of the work did not mean it is invalid, and they considered that environmental changes to produce congenial space were important. I wonder, however, if there is inherent bias in the appreciative enquiry model, as it directs partners in the programme to identify and assert positive outcomes. On the other hand, it shapes the ethos of a project. This is tricky.

The Invest to Save report has useful findings and motivational ideas, but there are gaps in structure and content, and the transformational model it follows seems overly complex. It is strong on identifying impacts on individuals, but there is almost no consideration of effects on groups and communities, which its holistic model might point towards. The report cites the public health White Paper *Choosing Health*[58] as the background context to the study, suggesting that the report would relate findings to how arts motivate healthy choices, but by the end it seems to shift more to therapeutic effects in institutional settings, even though NHS facilities have a growing public health dimension.

The report's findings provide some useful evidence, even if the 'standard' tools used (the General Health Questionnaire[59] and the Hospital Anxiety and Depression Scale[60]) are problematic for arts aims. It should have been acknowledged that the report's sample was limited as regards statistical significance, especially on job-satisfaction issues, where only a handful of staff were sampled but a control model was used. There was also a bias in the sample – 98% of people were white and 59% were over 55. The projects that were studied tell us some things about certain demographic groups but can only partially relate to population health and health inequalities issues addressed in *Choosing Health*.

Another focused arts programme to test a transformational model took place at Upstream Healthy Living Centre in Devon. Upstream is one of only five 'pathfinder' healthy living centres in the UK, and it has placed arts prominently in its programme and ethos. It undertook evaluation of its arts interventions with elderly people in 2005, combining qualitative and quantitative measures in an action research programme conducted by Mid Devon Primary Care Trust and Peninsula Medical School.[61]

The study surveyed 271 participants, 177 of whom took part in a mentored arts or social activity programme. Many participants were identified as socially isolated and/or depressed, and 19% were direct referrals from GPs. The most widely reported benefit was the social interactions occurring *around* the activities. Of the participants, 20–30% showed dramatic improvement in mood and 80–90% reported some benefit. A strong factor in this was the clients' perspective that services were tailored for their needs. The study used the York SF-12 questionnaire[62] as the main measurement tool but with an aim to translate these results into quality-adjusted life years (QALYs) for cost-benefit analysis. The study combined social identity theory (SIT) with self-concept theory (SCT), and it states:

> The central premise of SIT is that the more an individual identifies with a group, the more self-representations become intertwined with group defini-tions. SCT tells us that social self-representations are a crucial component of human self-concept (the sum of mental representations about the self), which when evaluated (positively or negatively) form the basis of self-esteem. The promotion of new, positive social /group identities (social participation) is therefore likely to affect individual self-concept and self-esteem in impor-tant ways. Self-esteem is a central pillar of mental health and psychological well-being, and self-representation and self-evaluation have a moderating role in emotional health (another crucial premise of self-concept theory). Having new socially meaningful roles therefore increases the opportunities for self-esteem to be enhanced, resulting in increased emotional health and well being.[63]

In both this study and Invest to Save, there is a tendency in the text to suggest that if A happens, the result is B leading to C, because the qualitative research is informed by the ideal world of a 'transformational' model. These studies tend to bypass variables and rush to conclusions in efforts to prove the creative flow of a diagram. This is a pity, because through their empathic observations of process they touch upon what may be at the core of this work, as I shall explain in my final chapter.

A more measured approach to testing a 'theory of change' can be found in research commissioned by the Department of Health and the Department for Culture, Media and Sport.[64] The two-year study, carried out by researchers at Anglia Ruskin University and the University of Central Lancashire, aimed to identify appropriate indicators and outcome measures from arts interventions in a range of mental health settings and to develop and implement an evaluation framework.

Indicators of improved mental health were identified as increased levels of mental well-being, decreased mental distress, reduced levels of primary and secondary care service use and reduced medication. Indicators of increased social inclusion were higher levels of social contact likely to build bonding and bridging social capital, reduced levels of perceived stigma and discrimination and higher levels of engagement in employment and education. 'Distance travelled' indicators, measuring empowerment, included increased levels of confidence and self esteem, enjoyment of arts participation, learning/skills gained and pride in work produced.

The research developed a combination of its own and existing measures for an outcomes study across 22 projects, at baseline and after six months, assessing levels of mental health, social inclusion and empowerment through a framework that attempted to reflect the 'distance travelled' through a project by each participant. Six projects were also selected for qualitative case study.

Triangulation of results suggested that there was very strong evidence for empowerment, with less strong evidence for improvement in mental health and social inclusion, though the report concluded that the results justify support for arts in mental health work from statutory services. It also cautions that arts provision for people with mental health needs is not a case of 'one size fits all', and this has to be taken into account when designing projects.

The qualitative study concluded that it is not meaningful to attempt to measure changes in medication and levels of service use, but the contribution of arts participation to recovery is worth pursuing. Arts should not be reduced to just individual psychological and therapeutic benefits, as user-led notions of recovery place the activity in a social rather than a medical model. It is not necessarily all about medication, symptoms and services post-discharge; it is also about individuals beginning able to live the kind of lives they want to live. Key common themes in recovery include:
➤ finding hope, meaning, purpose and value
➤ finding new coping mechanisms
➤ developing new identities within and beyond mental health.

It is precisely these aspects that arts in mental health projects seem to tackle best, yet these are particularly hard to standardise and measure.

It is impressive that this first nationwide study has attempted to engage with the complexity of arts in mental health and has successfully brought a large number of projects into a common evaluation framework that allows statistical significance to be drawn from a wide range of identified outcomes. There are some problems, however, in both methodology and results. The authors of the study have acknowledged, in a separate review article, a need to distinguish between psychological and social empowerment, clarifying whether outcomes are indicative only of passive adjustment or whether they constitute genuine social empowerment.[65] This could also prove useful in helping distinguish between the approaches of arts therapies and participatory arts.

The research's qualitative case studies adopt an interpretative stance that seems at odds with the highly rigorous approach to data in the quantitative analysis, suggesting that combined measures for this work may produce perspectives that are difficult to reconcile. In the survey results on the empowerment issue, it is interesting that a question about 'mutual aid' did not score to statistical significance. If it had, it would have had bearing on demonstrating social empowerment. Yet projects scored highly on that question at baseline. Presumably one possible reason is that participatory arts are the core of the activity, so it would have been useful to consider how similar/dissimilar the six projects were, what affect their participatory ethos had on participants from the outset and whether communal as well as individualised outcomes were realised. Retaining this contextual information on projects in the study might also have strengthened data on social inclusion outcomes.

## A SOCIAL-MAPPING MODEL

A common weakness in projects that test a 'transformational' model is that although these projects are community-based, they are precisely targeted to specific groups, so it is difficult to generalise results as applicable to communities as a whole. A social-mapping approach could help gather data from a more diverse sample of participants. It may also prove worthwhile to spend more time analysing concepts of community well-being generated by arts participation before attempting to demonstrate them.

What I think has been groundbreaking research in this respect is an evaluation study carried out over three years by the Globalism Institute in Melbourne, with VicHealth, of four community arts programmes in both urban and outback Victoria.[66] The study's starting point is recognition that well-being has become a preoccupation of health promotion agencies, and it distinguishes between individualised well-being and social patterns of well-being through which sustainability is seen primarily as a process of support and interaction assisted by critical reflection. It advocates participant-based evaluation, and it considers that too much focus to date on indicators has led to over-instrumentalised approaches that have overlooked longer-term assessment of benefit. Instead the study uses a process it terms 'social mapping' to describe a combination of quantitative and qualitative data collection and analysis, including photo-narrative methods. This generates narratives of meaning that are complex but give depth rather than a shallow breadth of short-term indicators.

This study advocates building separate projects into research programmes, but it is cautious about using a diagram-driven transformation model, because 'a crucial strength of the arts is that they can have a multitude of overlapping and interlocking purposes and it is impossible to represent this adequately with a two-dimensional map or matrix.'[67] It sees a need to identify wider public outcomes than just event-specific ones, and it concludes that its research data suggests that social inclusion appears to be affected in a meaningful way only through long-term ongoing involvement in community arts.

The study has a good sense of how artists approach their practice, recognising that some projects may be purposefully short-term or may dissipate their energy but the need is to reinvent and regenerate. It notes that artists stress the need for authentic engagement and the use of local stories and argues this must not be watered down by over-attention to social inclusion as the goal. The socio-economic status of community artist affects recognition of the importance of their work and its research.

The emphasis on the relational aspects of arts activity suggests to the report's authors that 'agency' is a better term for encapsulating the fostering of self-determination in community arts: 'Our intention in using the term agency over autonomy is to emphasise the irretrievably social character of such activity. Agents are always bound into social relationships, mores and commitments which both enable and constrain action.'[68]

The report even suggests that potential benefit can still be sensed in non-participation. While recognising the need to target activity and provide participants with a quality experience of arts development, it also sees importance in 'avowal', meaning the wider recognition in a community that something positive is happening even though you might not take part in it. It identifies a phenomenon it terms 'abstracted inclusion', where one may wish to contribute something to a community but not directly take part in its activities. These subtleties of (non-)engagement are also important to respecting difference while building social cohesion. The report concludes that, on a global level, the issue of community sustainability is now as crucial as confronting environmental concerns.

How far should the vanguard of arts in health move into a community development arena? As multi-sector collaborations increasingly assist the delivery of arts in community health and theoretical disciplines converge to examine its effects, the field is establishing a research agenda around a social model of health. This must not, however, diminish the ability it also has to illuminate and inform the work of medical and health professionals. Investigation into therapeutic effects and the reliable attribution of benefit for healthcare from the arts should continue. There is otherwise a danger of over-generalising health gain from sustainable development and social inclusion outcomes. Much of this work originated in the UK within primary care, and that is where public health's on-the-ground services are now based. In future what could help maintain a balance between sociological and clinical investigation into community arts would be a closer alliance between the diverse practice of the arts in health field and the sharpening vision of medical humanities, as envisioned in my final chapter. Such an alliance could help overcome many of the difficulties and dilemmas that have so far hampered the development of a credible evidence base for the effectiveness of participatory arts on community health.

## REFERENCES

1 Feynman RP. *The Meaning of It All*. London: Allen Lane; 1998. p. 28.
2 Matarasso F. *Use or Ornament? The social impact of participation in the arts*. Stroud: Comedia; 1997. p. 68.
3 Wilson M. *Health is for People*. London: Darton, Longman and Todd; 1975. p. 2.
4 Pirsig R. *Lila: an inquiry into morals*. New York: Bantam; 1991. pp. 126–7.
5 Cleveland Arts. *Articulate*. Middlesbrough: Cleveland Arts; 2002. p. 23.
6 Angus J. *A Review of Evaluation in Community Based Arts in Health*. London: Health Development Agency; 2002. Available at: www.dur.ac.uk/resources/cahhm/reports/CAHHM%20for%20HDA%20J%20Angus.pdf (accessed 3 January 2009).
7 Hacking S, Secker J, Spandler H, *et al*. *Mental Health, Social Inclusion and the Arts*. London: National Social Inclusion Programme; 2007.
8 Staricoff R. *Arts in Health: a review of the medical literature (research report 36)*. London: Arts Council England; 2004.
9 Wilson J. *Your Health and the Arts: a study of the association between arts engagement and health*. London: Arts Council England; 2005.
10 Ibid. p. 77.
11 Byrgen LO, Konlaan BB, Johanssson SE. Swedish interview survey of living conditions. *BMJ*. 1996; **313**: 1577–80.
12 Health Promotion Evaluation Unit. *Survey on Recreation and Health 1992–2006 Vol. 2: participation in the arts*. Perth: University of Western Australia; 2007.
13 Health Promotion Evaluation Unit. *Sponsorship Monitor Evaluation Results 2006/07*. Perth: University of Western Australia; 2007.
14 Putland C. Lost in Translation: the question of evidence linking community-based arts and health promotion. *J Health Psychol*. 2008; **13**(2): 265–76.
15 Macnaughton RJ, White M, Stacy R. Researching the Benefits of Arts in Health. *Health Educ*. 2005; **105**(5): 332–9.
16 Angus J, White M. *Arts and Adult Mental Health Literature Review*. Durham: University of Durham (CAHHM); 2003.

17 Smith T. *Common Knowledge: an evaluation of sorts.* Durham: University of Durham (CAHHM); 2003. p. 23.

18 Kagan C. Temporary weblog entry on Arts Council England arts debate at www.artscouncil.org.uk (accessed 15 September 2007).

19 Dileo C, Bradt J. *Medical Music Therapy: a meta-analysis and agenda for future research.* Cherry Hill, NJ: Jeffrey Books; 2005.

20 Moriarty G. *Sharing Practice: a guide to self-evaluation for artists, arts organisations and funders working in the context of social exclusion.* London: Arts Council England; 2003.

21 Everitt A, Hamilton R, White M, editors. *Arts, Health and Community: a study of five arts in community health projects.* Durham: University of Durham (CAHHM); 2003.

22 Wallerstein N. *What is the Evidence on Effectiveness of Empowerment to Improve Health?* Copenhagen: WHO Europe Health Evidence Network; 2006. p. 20.

23 Francis P. Participatory Development at the World Bank: the primacy of process. In: Cooke B, Kathari U, editors. *Participation: the new tyranny.* London: Zed Books; 2001.

24 Coote A, Allen J, Woodhead D. *Finding Out What Works: understanding complex, community-based initiatives.* London: King's Fund; 2004.

25 Ibid. p. 4.

26 Ibid. p. 50.

27 Mason J. *Qualitative Researching.* London: Sage; 2002.

28 Launer J. Narrative and mental health in primary care. In: Greenhalgh T, Hurwitz G, editors. *Narrative Based Medicine.* London: BMJ Books; 1998. p. 93.

29 Smith R. Spend (slightly) less on health and more on the arts. *BMJ.* 2002; **325:** 1432–3.

30 HM Treasury. *The Green Book: appraisal and evaluation in central government.* London: Stationery Office; 2003.

31 Kelly G, Muers S. *Creating Public Value: an analytical framework for public service reform.* London: Strategy Unit of the Cabinet Office; 2001.

32 Lidstone G. Evaluating arts education programmes. In: Cowling J, editor. *For Art's Sake? Society and the arts in the 21st century.* London: ippr; 2004. p. 53.

33 The Council for Museums, Archives and Libraries. *Learning Impact Research Project.* Leicester: University of Leicester; 2002.

34 Power M. The World Health Organization WHOQOL-100. *Health Psychol.* 1999; **18**(5): 495–505.

35 *The Warwick-Edinburgh Mental Well-being Scale.* Available at: www.healthscotland.com/documents/1467.aspx (accessed 30 July 2008).

36 CORE System. Available at: www.coreims.co.uk (accessed 6 August 2008).

37 Hacking, Secker, Spandler, *et al.*, op. cit.

38 Health Education Authority. *Art for Health: a review of practice in arts-based projects that impact on health and well-being.* London: Health Education Authority; 2000.

39 Argyle M. Sources of satisfaction. In: Christie I, editor. *The Good Life: Demos collection number 14.* London: Demos; 1998.

40 Matarasso F, Chell J. *Vital Signs: mapping community art in Belfast.* Stroud: Comedia; 1998.

41 Campbell C, Wood R, Kelly M. *Social Capital and Health.* London: Health Education Authority; 1999.

42 Hacking, Secker, Spandler, *et al.*, op. cit.

43 Pawson R, Tilley N. *Realistic Evaluation*. London: Sage Publications; 1997.

44 Brice-Heath S, Wolf S. *Visual Learning in the Community School*. London: Creative Partnerships; 2004.

45 Brice-Heath S. *Artshow: a resource guide*. Washington: Partners For Liveable Communities; 1999.

46 Centre for Leisure and Sport Research. *Count Me In: the dimensions of social inclusion through culture and sport*. Leeds: Leeds Metropolitan University; 2002.

47 Ibid. p. 84.

48 Centre for Cultural Policy Research. *Quality of Life and Well-being: measuring the benefits of culture and sport*. Edinburgh: Scottish Executive; 2006.

49 Everitt, Hamilton, White, editors, op. cit.

50 Bhandari BB. *Participatory Rural Appraisal*. Arlington: Institute for Global Environmental Strategies; 2003. Available at: www.iges.or.jp/en/pub/eLearning/water demo/bhandari_m4.pdf (accessed 6 August 2008).

51 Francis P, op. cit. p. 83.

52 Ibid. p. 85.

53 Kelaher M, Berman N, Joubert L, *et al. Methodological Approaches to Evaluating the Impact of Community Arts on Health*. Melbourne: University of Melbourne; 2007.

54 Nolan E. *Performance Indicators as an Evaluation Technique for Arts in Health Projects*. Waterford: Waterford Institute of Technology; 2004.

55 Matarasso F. *Defining Values: evaluating arts programmes*. Stroud: Comedia; 1996. p. 7.

56 Kilroy A, Garner C, Parkinson C, *et al. Towards Transformation: exploring the impact of culture, creativity and the arts on health and well-being*. Manchester: Manchester Metropolitan University; 2007.

57 Keyes CLM, Shmotkin D, Ryff CD. Optimizing well-being: the empirical encounter of two traditions. *J Pers Soc Psychol*. 2002; **82**: 1007–22.

58 Department of Health. *Choosing Health: making healthier choices easier* [White Paper]. London: Department of Health, 2004.

59 Goldberg D. The General Health Questionnaire. Available at: www.gp-training.net/protocol/docs/ghq.doc (accessed 6 August 2008).

60 Available at: www.refhelp.scot.nhs.uk/dmdocuments/HADS_scoring_sheet.pdf (accessed 6 August 2008).

61 Greaves C, Farbus L. *Upstream Healthy Living Centre: research on the processes and outcomes of an intervention to address social isolation in the elderly*. Exeter: Peninsula Medical School; 2005.

62 Available at: www.crufad.com/phc/sf-12.htm (accessed 14 August 2008).

63 Greaves, Farbus, op. cit. p. 9.

64 Hacking, Secker, Spandler, *et al.*, op. cit.

65 Secker J, Spandler H, Hacking S. Empowerment and arts participation for people with mental health needs. *J Public Ment Health*. 2008; 6(4): 14–23.

66 Mulligan M, Humphery K, James P, *et al. Creating Community: celebrations, arts and wellbeing within and across local communities*. Melbourne: Globalism Institute RMIT; 2006.

67 Ibid. p. 31.

68 Ibid. p. 133.

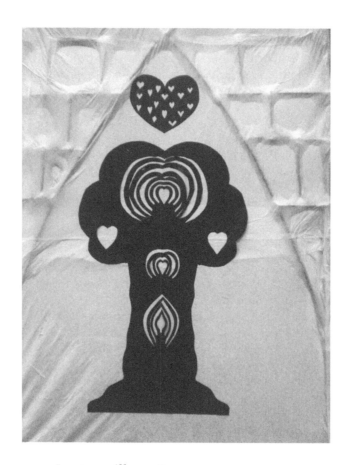

Lantern silhouette. PHOTO: MARY ROBSON

# CHAPTER 9

# Are we there yet? The destination of arts in community health

The emergence of a new culture is rarely if ever the result of a conscious choice with a definite goal in mind.

René Dubos, *So Human an Animal*[1]

When I began to work in the arts in health field in the late 1980s, the few examples that could be found of established programmes were hospital-based. This set the precedent that arts in health should look to develop dialogue between the arts and the medical sector. A burden was placed on the arts – often as a result of confusing them with art therapies – to demonstrate they have a viable role in treatment and recuperation and to provide evidence of benefit.

Delivery of the work, however, has suggested that a more effective role lies in creating environmental improvements, whether physical or sensory, that can indirectly influence a sense of wellness, and in building morale in the work-force by nurturing a visible culture of healthcare. As the field has diversified and extended into primary care and community health, it has become clear to me that the dialogue needed here is in fact between the health and education sectors, with arts as a creative medium for the exploration and expression of that dialogue.

As arts in community health is essentially a grassroots movement, this book has focused on the distinctive character of practice and looked at how learning in this field can be shared at both a local and international level. The development of the work has proceeded organically and often without 'a definite goal in mind'. Consequently, those delivering or supporting arts in community health have felt that a strategic vision, with the right incentives to forge network connections, needs to emerge quickly for fear that in a few years all of this pioneering work could dissipate.

Hard evidence from cultural research into the impact of arts engagement on individual and population health, however, is still limited, and this is stalling decision-makers. What could be persuasive evidence from epidemiology on the importance to health of social status and self-esteem (where arts participation could demonstrate a useful role) has not so far included consideration of how a thriving culture might mitigate the effects of health inequalities. Meanwhile, social capital theorists argue a need for integration through culture but fall short on methods for reliably and sensitively measuring key issues of how autonomy and quality are generated out of civic engagement.

Civil society may be in decline in respect to its traditional infrastructure, as Putnam suggests,[2] but technology has changed the protocols of human association. This is evident in the virtual communities that thrive through the internet. In contradiction to Illich's tenet[3] that post-war medicine has come to disempower people's relationship with their health, web-based communication around health issues and consumer power are growing, and this impacts on clinical consultation. The changes in culture that result from health becoming increasingly related to personal well-being and capacity for living are prompting calls for a new research agenda to emerge from a patient-centred model for health. RPN Rainsberry has argued that this has to allow for 'subjective science' grounded in the psychosocial aspects of illness.[4] It requires a shift in moral and political values, not just in scientific thinking. The problem is that primary care research has tended to be weighted to the objective model through epidemiology alone. As Rainsberry asserts:

> We need research of the imagination, research that takes its cue from an experience of illness rather than a description . . . it is anecdotal, subjective and fictional to some extent. This is the only way in which the value questions and issues that must guide family medicine research will emerge.[5]

This view has helped give rise to the current interest in medical education in narrative-based medicine, which is based on the interpretation of illness, not just its investigation. In this approach, the equity of the patient-doctor relationship is essential. Narrative-based medicine sets a patient-centred agenda and is sensitive to an oral tradition that medicine has declined to address since the rise of the techno-medical model. Trisha Greenhalgh and Brian Hurwitz observe that:

> The notion of interpretation (the discernment of meaning) is a central concern of philosophers and linguists, but it is a concept with which doctors are often unfamiliar, and hence uncomfortable. At its most arid, modern medicine lacks a metric for existential qualities such as inner hurt, despair, hope, grief and moral pain which frequently accompany, and often indeed constitute, the illnesses

from which people suffer. Narratives, in expressing our own attempts to make sense of our lives, usually presuppose causation.[6]

This is where medicine can become confounded by a complexity that lies beyond the physiological. A natural ally for arts in health in the exploration of this complexity is the field of medical humanities, particularly in its concern with the quality of communication between the medical practitioner and the public. It is here that a dialogue between medicine and arts could be of real purpose, evolving at a philosophical level that can shape creative enquiry rather than at a clinical level requiring physiological proof of benefit.

Iona Heath argues the need for a balance of emotional engagement and objective judgement in medical consultations with patients, drawing an analogy here with wave/particle theory.[7] She cites the centrality of social inclusion policy, because if public health perspectives are to address health inequalities, they need to focus particularly on the most vulnerable and marginalised individuals. Looking at impacts of low status on health, she goes on to say that a greater sense of social control, allowing freer rein for individual moral autonomy, promotes health and prevents illness and disease. She advocates more empathic consultation:

> In interrogation the interrogator frames questions entirely within the context of his or her own world view; whereas in engaging in a genuine dialogue, the listener attempts, through imagination, to move into the contextual horizon of the other's world.[8]

This is a skill that is often highly developed in artists, actors, musicians, poets and storytellers. There is growing evidence that creative empathy is intuitively applied in the human brain in consequence of it being hard-wired for social intelligence.[9] This is not only a phenomenon of neuroscience; it is also observable in culture.

Rainsberry's call for 'research of the imagination' is an exciting way forward for multidisciplinary investigation into the impact of creativity and reciprocity on health. There is an important role here for medical humanities in bridging science and arts discourses. In a 2008 submission to the Wellcome Trust, my research centre, CAHHM at Durham University, identified four thematic enquiries for the medical humanities to engage in, as follows:

1  to understand, challenge and seek to reconcile the divergence between scientific and experiential accounts of human nature, health and flourishing
2  to understand how to reduce or dissolve the harmful effects that this divergence has upon clinical healthcare and health policy
3  to pursue an intellectually coherent incorporation of humanities perspectives and understandings within clinical healthcare

4   to promote, within the bio-scientific understanding of human nature and flourishing, a recognition of the virtues of humanities' understanding – and vice versa.

To test hypotheses arising from these enquiries, CAHHM's outreach work has established links with projects in schools, hospitals, prisons and communities around the UK and internationally in which creative activities are integral to health promotion and well-being. Receiving a major award from the Wellcome Trust spurred CAHHM to re-name itself from 2009 as the Centre for Medical Humanities (or CMH). At the forefront of CMH work in the next five years is the aim to select a 'pathway' group of projects through which to assess public engagement ideas around health and medicine and their impact. Arts practitioners will be key collaborators in these 'pathway' projects. Collaborations such as those between CMH and primary schools in areas of high deprivation, for example, both help the teaching staff develop concepts of what makes a school 'flourishing' and help CMH reflect on its own ideas and processes in conducting action-based research.

CMH recognises that medical humanities may be better positioned than arts practice to be at the forefront of a debate with clinical healthcare professions. CMH's thematic inquiries in medical humanities will nevertheless extend into environments and situations where arts are being practically applied to health issues, and so these inquiries can assist the development of research-guided arts practice. The two fields find common ground in the nature of communication around health in both rational and experiential domains. Through medical humanities, future investigation into the benefits of arts in health could extend into assessing its impact on the practice of medicine and healthcare as well as its effects on patients and communities. This cross-disciplinary research will also have an important role in identifying and exploring ethical issues around the engagement of artists with communities on health issues, thereby assisting the development of good practice.[10] This is one university research organisation's sense of the destination of arts in community health within an academic framework. It helps to fulfil its mission and remit as a research centre uniquely spanning arts in health and medical humanities, but CMH is aware it is having to act in a policy vacuum as regards the arts field.

So what happened to an arts-led strategy? What could we have won? Arts Council England's national strategy for arts in health, which was in preparation from 2005–07, intended to focus mainly on ACE's own functions, funding systems and client base and to look at how encouragement and support for arts in health activity could be built into these. ACE regional offices were asked to facilitate cross-departmental meetings to consider how arts in health could be built into individual officers' portfolios, and indications from early meetings showed this to be a constructive way forward to maximise the arts system's resources. ACE analysed the frequency and success rate of arts in health applications to its Grants for the Arts scheme, looking at why any previous applications may have failed. To improve communication between the art form and development departments of ACE regional offices, it was proposed that art form officers would be asked to comment on all applications received by the development department for arts in health projects.

In ACE's social inclusion portfolio, arts in health sat alongside arts in criminal justice and the Creative Partnerships arts in education initiative, and this was useful at the time. They were all working to present the arts not as a diversionary palette but as a social platform exploring solutions for improvement in life prospects for individuals at risk. They also dealt with similar issues around evaluation, attempting to devise appropriate methodologies to assess impact and benefits.

ACE also examined how its support for touring work could be extended to include exhibitions and performances in healthcare buildings. More opportunities for arts in health could be identified in major development initiatives such as New Audiences, Creative Partnerships, and Artsmark, which singled out venues and organisations with a track record of presenting high-quality arts activity.

Significant improvement in the advocacy and promotion of arts in health activity might be had if ACE were to provide the kind of marketing support it gave to its cultural diversity scheme – which could find a ready parallel in social marketing schemes in the health sector. ACE's national strategy was concerned with making its infrastructure more favourable for arts in health, and the regional action plans focused on organic and bottom-up development through partnerships. They were to develop in parallel, each guiding the other as to where activities and resources might be best placed. With hindsight, however, it seems each plan misguidedly confused strategic planning with effective advocacy, resulting in a watered down publication.[11] ACE's more upbeat joint prospectus with the Department of Health[12] foundered because neither ACE nor NHS organisations were able to go forward on it because of a shortage of resources and a fear of media backlash.

At the time, this was a big disappointment to the arts in health field, but it may have been a blessing that the field escaped being circumscribed by official sanction. There was little indication that ACE had the commitment, let alone the resources, to shape a development strategy for a complex and diverse field of practice that posed difficult questions about the role of subsidised arts. ACE's interim consultation report on the strategy[13] was too inward-looking, not recognising that the majority of arts in health activity was supported outside of the arts funding system and that what place the activity had within ACE's portfolio was of little consequence. Budgetary pressures meant that ACE was actually having to disinvest in its arts in health clients at that time. Worse still, by 2008, with arts budgets slashed to accommodate preparations for the 2012 Olympics, ACE's chief executive was prepared to state openly that arts in health was not a priority consideration.[14]

The lack of follow-up action on the Department of Health's review prompted a House of Lords debate on arts in health on 6 March 2008, in which Lord Haworth made an eloquent plea for 'political leadership' to be exerted in support of arts in health, but to no avail.[15] Then on 16 September 2008 the Secretary of State for Health Alan Johnson MP delivered an upbeat speech in support of arts in health, promising that the Department of Health would set up a unit to assist with advocacy and the identification of sources of support.[16] At time of writing, this unit has not yet materialised. Is there cause for concern here, or has one opportunity for a convergence of the arts and health sectors simply passed, and we must wait for the next one? With the sudden collapse, at least temporarily, of Arts Council support, and despite an abiding lack of formal leadership, I find myself little concerned about the strategy vacuum; arts in community health has always been a hybrid activity that finds its support outside mainstream budgets. On-the-ground experience has shown there is an entrepreneurial momentum to the development of the work, and continuing with an organic and opportunist growth may suit it better than a guiding external strategy. Whatever temporary funding difficulties are faced by individual practitioners, there is the inexorable motion of a growing traffic of ideas towards a common destination.

What I want to show in this final chapter is how different perspectives on issues central to arts in community health are starting to coalesce in a way that will guide mission and practice in arts in community health for years to come. I wish to highlight some of the things that several people from different professions said to me in preparation for this book (mostly in interviews conducted between 2006 and 2008), using their voices to provide commentary and insight, and hopefully offer some resolution of issues raised in previous chapters. I refer to these people in the professions/roles they held at the time of interview.

I believe that arts in community health has already gone beyond the issues that might formalise a structural partnership between the arts and health sectors. It has moved into the central arena of health policy in respect of Lord Darzi's 2008 review of the NHS, *High Quality Care For All*,[17] and its key concern to achieve an empowered workforce that can deliver quality health services reflecting public perception of what makes for a caring NHS. This goes beyond structural reforms to examine the very mission of the health service, and, as the NHS Confederation noted, it needs to be manifest both in directing skills and improving interpersonal relations on the ground: 'The local nature of delivery makes it very dependent on the quality of local leadership and is a very significant challenge'.[18] Kathryn Fitch, a freelance consultant working closely with one of the largest primary care trusts in the country in the north of England, offers an acute observation on how and where that challenge originates:

Our PCT has a vision that is good on principles and aspirations but may have more progress to make on how that translates into practice for staff, in terms of 'what does that mean in practice?' It seems that people at all levels of the organisation are finding it difficult to articulate what change might require and what it might look like, so development programmes are themselves suffering from this blight too. It may also be the case that the new PCT structure, in places, is not helping. The PCT senior managers are essentially over busy and have insufficient time to devote to the thinking around all of this and are busy producing lots of paper evidence that change is occurring when in fact it isn't very much – just lots of new language, a lot of paperwork and some small changes to practice. In the face of this overwhelming agenda, many staff shrink back to their perceived sphere of influence and sometimes even shrink within this to produce only what they must in relation to the 'paper evidence' game. Staff are therefore inevitably feeling pressured and in development terms probably just want to be told what to do. However, there is no way of being able to do that when everything is new – it's about supporting people to find their way towards some shared vision (which people are finding hard to paint). If ever there was a time for creative collaboration to come to the fore – it is now![19]

When I interviewed John Ashton, regional director of North West Public Health, he saw that such 'creative collaboration' needs to proceed politically out of a progressive coalition that includes artists, because there is 'a very clear value structure in that many of those who have gone through community arts as their training ground have then been able to go into areas of social policy and have a sense of what it is they can contribute without simply trying to be some sort of instrumental tool to whatever initiative is coming out of the health service', though he added pessimistically that 'it's the best of times, it's the worst of times. A lot of people who are in key positions to do anything about public health don't understand it. They are talking about public health as reductionist lifestyle interventions.'[20] Ashton explained to me that he quit his trained profession as a psychiatrist because he saw that individual therapy was inadequate to deal with the public health dimension of mental health, where:

you've got to come at it from a community solution. It's about understanding childhood and parenting, but also about support networks and communities. What I say to colleagues who trained with me and who spend their life dealing with individuals is if you've really become so dependent on your patients, do it one–two days a week. Spend the rest of your time working with head teachers, personnel managers and other 'people people', giving them the benefit of your advice and support to reach many more.[21]

Ashton softens the impact of Illich's 'limits to medicine' by recognising that participation in creative activity generates meaning whereby:

> If people made more sense of their health and illnesses, they might be less inclined to turn to health services, and live with the condition better rather than simply trying to get rid of it. The shared meanings possible in community arts practice may be the basis of a common pursuit of preventative health as a viable complement – if not alternative – to those reductionist lifestyle interventions.[22]

If the creative engagement of a preventative healthcare service were given room to prove its effectiveness, it may be more useful for therapy to withdraw from frontline service to a support role – and not just for the client. Availability of peer support and counselling for artists working in the field is an important issue, and it should be integral to their training in arts in community health. To combat the stress and emotional challenges that often accompany this kind of work, artists would benefit from the professional supervision that is a norm of art therapy practice. Should this also be offered to other professionals in the arts in health field – not just artists – it would serve the additional purpose of strengthening the fundamental relationships that underpin the work. Arts in health training courses need to link with placements in on-the-ground projects that are followed up with mentoring and supervision. CMH's artist/research associate Mary Robson has become a strong advocate of this approach, as she explains:

> The field of arts in health draws practitioners from many disciplines. As well as artists, there are health workers, educators, individuals, local authority personnel, voluntary sector workers who can all be involved. Relatively few have knowledge or experience of professional supervision or other support mechanisms as part of their working lives. It is not only freelance artists who may never have teachers; general practitioners, occupational therapists also – the list could go on and on. All come across challenging and demanding scenarios in their working lives. Individual and group supervision could prove a boon to an emergent field such as arts in health.
>
> Often project partners work together for a short time, sometimes in challenging circumstances. The learning points of the experience could be captured in planned, regular facilitated sessions that are guided by techniques of reflective practice. They would contribute to the development and evaluation of the project – for example, through openly contracting the partnership at the outset and course correction throughout the process. Whilst artists have been offered training in business techniques, few have the opportunity to access and afford personal management training. Short courses that look at achieving goals,

avoiding burn-out, managing conflicting priorities and balancing personal and professional commitments could be offered at a subsidised rate as part of a training and supervision programme.[23]

Hull's arts and health manager, Elaine Burke, formerly a trained art therapist, believes the emotional pressures can be circumscribed and resolved as well-managed operational issues, particularly if adequate resource is allocated to project planning so that a risk strategy can be embedded from the outset. Both she and Mary Robson are adamant that therapy has no place in the actual delivery of the work, because it is not issue-based and artists should be freed to 'deliver high-quality art intervention that is about helping people to get the best experience they can have.' Elaine is jointly employed by Hull's Community Mental Health Trust and Hull Primary Care Trust, and they have embraced arts in community health to the extent that their policy decisions routinely require consideration of whether there is an arts dimension. (If this had happened in Cork, it might have better sustained its programme after Capital of Culture.) Such a comprehensive approach to utilising the arts has significantly influenced service delivery in young people's mental health, for example. There are transparent directives in programme development, and projects are usually for a minimum of one year, with some of the youth-oriented work sustained now for nearly 10 years. As Burke explains:

> I usually write an outline document which comes out of our vision of what we understand is the focus of our work. Then I go around all the managers first; I do it top-down because with experience if you don't get the managers on board you can forget it. I then tweak the document in line with those discussions and then we go to the staff and all the staff tweak the document again and then we have our final document that we are working to. There is loads of flexibility. The aims of the project are in there, such as well-being, boosting self-confidence and esteem, but we also make it clear about copyright and consent; all those things are made crystal clear, along with management's responsibility. We set up all the operational stuff to deal with what can go wrong.[24]

There is a clarity of management process here that should be informing the characteristics of practice that I described in Chapter 3, and fostering ownership of innovation through consultation might counteract the entropy that Fitch has identified in her PCT. Unfortunately there are scarce examples yet of arts in health posts like Burke's that have been instigated internally by health trusts. Hull PCT has actively encouraged the work to go beyond providing instrumental interventions to address the big picture of a city's health – in the case of Hull, a city that badly needed to turn around its low ranking on health, education and socioeconomic indicators. Burke sees the success of the arts in health programme here as partly due to having everything to play for: 'I think the whole symbiosis between the art that we deliver in a healthcare context and the wider community out there and the arts infrastructure is really of interest because you start to pick out trends of change a lot better.'[25]

A health service perspective on what arts in health could be addressing was summed up for me in some off-the-record comments made by the chief executive of a strategic health authority:

> There is a history of arts in health strategies produced in the arts sector which have one thing in common – that the NHS doesn't know of them! The reality is that to shift from arts in health as a minority interest promoted only where there are local advocates to something more mainstream requires two things:
>
> One – The strategic thinking needs to be embedded in health priorities, with consideration of how that can in turn support arts priorities (not the other way round). Obvious opportunities exist in terms of supporting patient choice and patient-centred care, in delivering culturally sensitive services, in opening up NHS employment to new workforce, in the links between health services and local regeneration (seeing health facilities as community resources), in taking forward key parts of the public health agenda and in supporting the transition from hospital-based care to community care. The health service needs to understand better how this agenda supports them in achieving what they have to do.
>
> Two – We need an arts in health workforce. The difference made by an arts coordinator can be profound, especially when he or she is really aware of how the health service works, can work in an operational/managerial environment and knows how to access partnership resources, as well as being perhaps a creative artist. This needs training and development, and many health institutions are desperate for advice and support in this area but simply don't know where to start.

Professor Chris Drinkwater, head of the Primary Care Development Centre at University of Northumbria at Newcastle, also sees the appointment within health trusts of arts in health coordinators as crucial: 'GPs don't know what the alternatives [to medical intervention] are, and there isn't a portfolio – but it might be the arts in health coordinator who can say this is the range of options and the choices available.'[26] He argues that medical training needs to recognise public health as a people skill, because:

> Historically in the medical mind, public health has worked very well in terms of sanitation and infectious disease. But in terms of chronic disease it's far less effective, because that is about individual behaviour. If you are going to change individual behaviour, you need to engage with communities. Arts are a means

to engage people and create a dialogue about healthy choices in a social and more open model than the rather deterministic approaches that are top-down. My view would be that unless you get the community engagement, there's no point in one-to-one approaches and motivational interviewing.[27]

The specificity required of community engagement can pose complex challenges, as I learned from Beverley Healey, coordinator of Artscare's work at Mater Hospital in Belfast. In the past, the hospital's outreach arts programme has had to overcome sectarian division, and the notion of collective creativity has had to be carefully managed:

> Every two years I would try and do one major project that involves the Shankhill community. The community forum is run by the hospital and made up from different local groups, and that is where a lot of my starting points have come from. I see it as anybody who comes to the hospital is a community resource, but then you have got people who are inside and outside that community, and bringing the two sides together is what we are very interested in doing. If people have an issue with their hospital or community, it is almost the 'gestalt' thing as you get the sum of the parts when you bring the two communities together. Sectarianism has figured in this area quite strongly. But only once did it come up for us, when two Catholic schools were working with two Protestant schools and one group decided not to be part of it, so it was a bit unbalanced. I think the advantage of working in the hospital setting is that the community is mixed already and there is nothing that can be done about it. So this hospital is more neutral. Obviously in a lot of these projects people know that it involves working with other groups, but they do not necessarily meet the other groups either, so that would not cause a problem in that sense. Sometimes they do and then it can cause a problem.[28]

It is interesting that in a fractured community a healthcare facility can be regarded as a 'neutral' space. As I mentioned in my earlier account of Wrekenton lanterns, an arts in community health project can call a truce on local quarrels, or as in the case of CDP in Johannesburg, it can highlight social injustice. I suspect that projects that are genuinely empowering are likely to get to the crux of a community's problems as well as the problems of individuals.

For Alison Jones at Looking Well, empowerment can also be a slow, hidden and incremental process: 'It works through conversation, not through going to the doctor, where you don't have to take responsibility. We are enabling people to take the next small step all the time. Why is it that the small steps are so huge?' Yet when reflecting on her first residency at Dr Rigler's surgery in 1988, she notes how small interventions have lasting effects:

The things that came up in three to four days in his surgery waiting room we are still doing. The lantern procession, which was a way of engaging people in the community around primary care, has continued to happen. The health promotion stuff, the art posters giving health messages, has been seen as educative and good. The Meet-a-Mum group making cards for new babies sparks conversation and keeps going. Now we've spent 20 years doing it, and it feels like a real struggle trying to do it, yet the potential emerged really quickly, a bit like you do a sketch for a painting, but the production of the actual artwork takes many hours, and you can't get it right and you keep working at it. In a way that is all we are doing. I remember that for Dr Rigler, the ideal thing was to have an arts centre with a GP working in it; that would just be amazing. If health messaging were arts-based, it would be about the potential, what is possible. But yes, we have done it as nearly as we can, and we have struggled to make the connections with all those different partners.[29]

This takes me back to my own beginning at Dr Rigler's surgery, described in Chapter 1, and I can see that the real sustainability in this work has come from a realisation of potential – in oneself and others – more than from the administrative complexities of evidence-based strategy and fundraising. I have been pointed from the beginning towards a social vision of health, and I believe that is what we all want to see in practice.

Those paradoxically small but huge steps in social engagement that Alison Jones describes recognise that a motivation to healthier living proceeds from emotional response to reciprocal trust. Participatory arts can provide a channel for that to be celebrated, and artists working in this field consistently say that in facilitating this they want to make a difference to people's health because they genuinely care.

Artistic processes may confound the scrutiny of clinical examination, health policy review or evaluation technique, yet there is a benefit staring us intellectually in the face. The collective artwork comes to express temporarily an unconditional love within boundaried relationships. That is why participants instinctively so often 'get it' when professional observers may not. Their emotional response is the embodiment of meaning, and this phenomenon is now considered central to cognitive science. As the philosopher Mark Johnson asserts:

We need to know how emotion binds us to the world, helps appraise our experience, and makes action possible. One of the surprises in studying these deep, pre-reflective, emotion-laden, embodied aspects of meaning, conceptualisation and reason is that these turn out to be the very processes and elements traditionally explored in aesthetics and art theory.[30]

Although this phenomenon may not yet be proven to have a replicable thera-peutic effect on individual pathology, it does demonstrate how a benign communion around health awareness can be created and sustained in people and places. It affirms the popular commitment NHS founder Aneurin Bevan called for in public health that I referred to in my Introduction. I have experienced this 'commitment' in such diverse situations as candlelit walks around rundown housing estates in Gateshead, in the low moan of a cello playing in an intensive care unit, at a multimedia tea party in an old people's home in Cork and in the hive-like intimacy of the Siyazama doll-makers' village at Msinga.

So much of what I described earlier in the case examples constitutes new traditions and rites of transformation and transition. This suggests to me that an anthropological approach informed by medical humanities might be the most effective and sympathetic means of understanding the practice of arts in community health and assessing its benefits. It would permit researchers to immerse in the processes of how culture and well-being interrelate. Although individual arts in community health projects come to an end, there is rarely a final outcome from this relationship-based way of working, because it is per-petually ongoing. This is why the narrative of a project becomes so important; as Wilson asserted, health requires 'the languages of story, myth and poetry [to] also disclose its truth.'[31]

The travels I was able to undertake in preparing this book revealed that there is both common cause and cultural diversity in this creative commitment to improving public health. I believe arts in community health is going to venture deeper into building capacity in both health services and the communities they serve, and I anticipate it will work increasingly in an international dimension out of global concerns to improve preventative healthcare. This is a new field for arts development that can dynamically employ the dictum attributed to René Dubos of 'think globally, act locally'[32] and Bertolt Brecht's aphorism that 'every art contributes to the greatest art of all, the art of living'.[33]

Small steps can be huge when they affirm our interdependency for the health of both our communities and our world. As we circumnavigate the trade routes of community arts, health and education, the destination is less important than the journey of discovery. From the kaleidoscopic variety of professionals' comments that I have set out in this chapter, I perceive that there are policy drivers for arts in community health, even if they appear to be 'off-roading' because the work is still in an exploratory phase. The most potent contribution that this new field of arts practice can make is the revelation of just how creative community health can be.

## REFERENCES

1 Dubos R. *So Human an Animal.* London: Hart Davis; 1970. p. 102.
2 Putnam R. *Bowling Alone: the collapse and revival of American community.* New York: Simon and Schuster; 2000.
3 Illich I. *Limits to Medicine.* London: Boyars; 1976.
4 Rainsberry RPN. Values, paradigms and research in family medicine. *Fam Pract.* 1986; 3(4): 209–15.
5 Ibid. p. 214.
6 Greenhalgh T, Hurwitz B, editors. *Narrative Based Medicine.* London: BMJ Books; 1998. pp. 10–11.
7 Heath I. 'Uncertain clarity': contradiction, meaning and hope. *Brit J Gen Pract.* 1999; 49: 651–7.
8 Ibid. p. 655.
9 Goleman D. *Social Intelligence: the new science of human relationships.* London: Hutchinson; 2006.
10 Macnaughton J. Arts in health. In: Evans M, Ahlzen R, Heath I, *et al.*, editors. *Medical Humanities Companion Vol.1: Symptom.* Oxford: Radcliffe Publishing; 2008. pp. 71–85.
11 Arts Council England. *The Arts, Health and Wellbeing.* London: Arts Council England; 2007.
12 Arts Council England, Department of Health. *A Prospectus for Arts and Health.* London: Arts Council England; 2007.
13 Arts Council England. *Arts, Health and Well-being: a strategy for partnership.* London: Arts Council England; 2004.
14 Hebron D. *Open Letter to Alan Davey, Arts Council England.* London: London Arts in Health Forum; 25 June 2008.
15 House of Lords. Arts debate. London: Hansard; 6 March 2008.
16 Available at: www.lahf.com (accessed 3 January 2009).
17 Darzi A. *High Quality Care For All.* London: Department of Health; 2008. Available at: www.dh.gov.uk/en/Publicationsandstatistics/Publications/Publications PolicyAndGuidance/DH_085825 (accessed 3 January 2009).
18 NHS Confederation. *Briefing Number 168.* 2008. Available at: www.nhsconfed.org/ (accessed 6 August 2008).
19 Fitch K. e-mail correspondence. 24 September 2008.
20 Ashton J. Taped interview. 26 April 2006.
21 Ibid.
22 Ibid.
23 Robson M. *Professional and Personal Development for Arts in Health Practitioners.* Durham: University of Durham (CAHHM); 2002.
24 Burke E. Taped interview. 17 March 2005.
25 Ibid.
26 Drinkwater C. Taped interview. 19 July 2006.
27 Ibid.
28 Healey B. Taped interview. 22 August 2005.
29 Jones A. Taped interview. 18 January 2005.
30 Johnson M. Body meanings. *New Scientist.* 12 January 2008: 46–7.
31 Wilson M. *Health is for People.* London: Darton, Longman and Todd; 1975. p. 60.

32 Wikipedia. *René Dubos*. Available at: www.en.wikipedia.org/wiki/Rene_Dubos (accessed 6 August 2008).

33 Brecht B. Appendices to the 'Short Organum'. In: Willett J. *Brecht on Theatre: the development of an aesthetic.* New York: Hill and Wang; 1964. pp. 276–81. p. 276.

# Index